The Clay Cure

The Clay Cure

▲

Natural

Healing from

the Earth

▼

RAN KNISHINSKY

Healing Arts Press
Rochester, Vermont

Healing Arts Press
One Park Street
Rochester, Vermont 05767
www.gotoit.com

*Note to the reader: This book is intended as an informational guide. The
remedies, approaches, and techniques described herein are meant to
supplement, and not to be a substitute for, professional medical care or
treatment. They should not be used to treat a serious ailment without
prior consultation with a qualified health-care professional.*

Library of Congress Cataloging-in-Publication Data

Knishinsky, Ran, 1971–

      The clay cure : natural healing from the earth / Ran Knishinsky.
            p.   cm.
      Includes bibliographical references and index.
      ISBN 0-89281-775-5 (pbk. : alk. paper)
      1. Clay—Therapeutic use.   I. Title.
RM666.C545K55 1998   97-52081
615'.2—dc21   CIP

Printed and bound in Canada

10 9 8 7 6 5 4 3

Text design and layout by Kristin Camp
This book was typeset in Sabon

Healing Arts Press is a division of Inner Traditions International

There is enough for all. The earth is a generous mother; she will provide in plentiful abundance food for all her children if they will but cultivate her soil in justice and in peace.

Bourke Coekran

www.claycure.com

Since the first edition of *The Clay Cure* in 1998, I have received over a thousand letters, phone calls, and e-mails from clay eaters all over the globe. These clay eaters have asked me questions and have shared their fascinating pica stories with me. I still keep in touch with many of these people. But now I would like to see these disparate bands of global clay eaters grow into a community. In order to facilitate this bonding process, *The Clay Cure* Web site has been created!

The site is dedicated to all of the clay eaters in the world and those who are just curious about this fascinating practice. The site will be updated continuously and promises to be interesting, informative, and fun.

- Find current and accurate information on edible clay
- Learn about clay products in the natural foods marketplace
- Purchase edible clays & more
- Read success stories about clay cures from all over the world
- Share your own personal tales of clay with other online users
- Participate in the discussion forum
- Meet other users who eat clay and use clay
- Help to build the *Clay Cure Community*

Let's use www.claycure.com to create the #1 clay eating destination on the web!

Ran Knishinsky
May 20, 2001
Phoenix, Arizona

Contents

Acknowledgments

To Gil Gilly, who introduced me to my first heaping tablespoon of clay.

To Julie Ellefson, who first gave me the idea to write a book on eating clay.

To Dr. Don Burt, Professor of Geology at Arizona State University, for his time and input.

To Phil Stoller: "Ten tablespoons a day!"

To Dr. Alan Christianson, N.M.D. (Scottsdale, Arizona), for editing assistance and for valuable suggestions.

Gratitude to Jon Graham, Christine Sumner, Anna Chapman, and the entire staff of Inner Traditions.

And special thanks most of all to Robin Straus, my literary agent, for her ongoing patience and support.

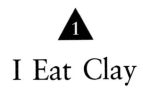

I Eat Clay

In the beginning God gave to every people a cup of clay, and from this cup they drank their life.

Native American Proverb

I have been eating dirt every day for the past six years. On purpose. It's a part of my diet. I never skip a day without eating clay. I may skip my vitamins and I may go without eating my vegetables, but I will never forget to take my clay. Sound funny? Probably, but I'm not the only one. Over two hundred cultures worldwide eat dirt on a daily basis.

The dirt of choice for many is clay. In India, some pour tea into new-formed clay teacups, drink the tea, then eat the cups. In South America, some cultures mix clay with honey and sugar as a sweet dessert, to be eaten after meals. In Europe, clay is sold for its gastrointestinal benefits and its purification properties.

We have long heard of people eating clay, known as either geophagy (pronounced gee-off-uh-gee) or pica. *Taber's Cyclopedic Medical Dictionary* defines geophagy as "a condition in which the patient eats inedible substances, such as chalk or earth." And it defines pica as "a perversion of appetite with

1

craving for substances not fit for food, such as clay, ashes or plaster. Condition seen in pregnancy, chlorosis (iron deficiency)." This craving may not be perverted at all, but makes sense when you know what clay contains and what it does for the body. It has been credited with improving the health of many people suffering from a wide range of illnesses. These include constipation, diarrhea, anemia, chronic infections, skin ailments such as eczema and acne, heavy-metal poisoning, exposure to pesticides and other toxins, arthritis, and stress. Whether clay is considered a substance not suited for eating really depends on where you travel on the globe.

WHY I STARTED EATING CLAY

I was first introduced to clay eating after a strange growth popped up on the back of my wrist. At the time, I didn't give it much thought so I ignored the problem, thinking it would go away, but the opposite happened—the lump grew larger in size. When it became a real interference, I had no choice but to get the bump checked out. My doctor diagnosed it as a "ganglion cyst," a cystic tumor usually connected with a joint or tendon.

"In the old days," he said, "they called it a 'Bible cyst.' That's because they used to smash the growth with a Bible to get rid of it."

He held my hand to the desk and showed me how it was done. "Now, however, we do surgery. The alternative isn't much better but it gets the job done."

"What do you recommend?" I asked.

His eyes lit up and he smiled. "Whichever one you like best."

Both answers to the problem sounded unappealing. I left the office and didn't bother to schedule another appointment.

When I got home, I took out my medical books and read fervently on ganglion cysts. I was hoping to discover some kind of reason why they occur. The doctor told me it was due to shock or trauma to the wrist, but somehow that answer didn't seem to fit right. The medical books made it clear that surgery was the only option available, other than waiting. And I had already waited six months without any definite progress. If I chose surgery, it would only treat the problem, not cure it. The cyst could always grow back, maybe bigger than before.

At my wits' end, I ran to the local health food store and met with the store owner. After I had related my experience to him, he explained that the cyst was not the result of shock to the wrist but was due to the buildup of poisons that had crystallized in the joint area. He grabbed a jar full of earth from his shelf and handed it to me.

"I recommend you eat clay," he said.

"Dirt?" I barked.

"Not any kind of dirt," he laughed. "A very special dirt."

"You mean eat it, like put it in my mouth?"

"Yes."

I wasn't averse to the idea of eating clay. I used to do it as a kid, sometimes eating charcoal or chalk. I had also heard of people who eat clay for medical purposes. Local magazines and newspapers always had an article here and there on clay eating. In fact, Pliny the Elder devoted an entire chapter of his "Natural History" to the many uses of clay. The practice was not limited to a tiny group by any means.

"Okay," I replied.

No sooner had I begun eating the clay day in and day out than within a period of two months, the growth shrank till it was completely gone. I couldn't believe my eyes. I showed my family the results—what was now a normal-looking wrist. My father attributed the disappearance of the cyst to coincidence. My mother claimed it was bound to go on its own anyway. Nobody cared to know the truth—it seemed too simple.

I, on the other hand, was astounded. Who would have thought that I could be healed by dirt! For the last couple of months, I had been dealing with a problem whose cure was right in my own backyard.

NATURAL MEDICINE

In the not too distant past, many people relied on natural medicine for minor ailments and chronic problems. There were no "miracle drugs," just old-fashioned home remedies. When you were sick, grandma made a batch of chicken soup and loaded you up with cod liver oil. Every family had bits and pieces of home doctoring knowledge. It was essential to life.

Natural medicines are pure medicines that accelerate our body's healing process to restore a healthy balance; they help us take care of ourselves. The more we listen to our bodies and the symptoms of our ailments, the more responsibility we can take for our health.

It makes sense to use the safe and effective remedies available to us. In light of modern medical knowledge, who would not take something as simple as an herb or a spoonful of dirt if they knew it would drastically help the situation—not to mention the possibility of avoiding side effects so often associated with conventional chemically created drugs? Home remedies will always have a place at the bedside, treating human aches and pains.

Folk remedies have made valuable contributions to scientific medicine. Many drugs and over-the-counter medications owe their existence to nature. For instance, white willow was one of the original sources of salicin, the chemical that led to the introduction of aspirin. And kaolin, a mineral clay, has been used valuably by the pharmaceutical industry in the form of Kaopectate to relieve intestinal diarrhea and distress.

The fundamental objective of natural medicines, as in clay, is to assist the body in working properly—to help the body help itself. Clay is not a quick cure for any disease. It is, however, especially suited to dealing with chronic complaints. Clay, given in small doses, is slow in effect, but the slow process evokes a more definite and radical cure than other supposed "quick-fix" medications.

In the past few years, scientific research has revealed some of the magic behind the workings of clay. This helps us to better understand its physiological actions, namely why clay is so effective in promoting and maintaining health. Yet, for all the scientific analysis done so far, we still don't know why or how clay exactly works. Apparently, like so many other things in the universe, nature keeps her work a secret. Consequently, it is up to us to learn how to use these natural gifts in a wise and intelligent manner.

OUR STATE OF HEALTH CARE

Modern health care, with its great contribution to emergency care and diagnostics, has done little to effectively prevent degenerative disease. The amount of arthritis, digestive disturbances, hypersensitivity conditions, allergies, cardiovascular disease, and nervous and mental disturbances that we witness today continues to increase.

Approximately seven million people in this country are afflicted with arthritis. Cancer claimed nearly one-half million lives in 1994, making it the second most common cause of death. Also, in 1994 heart disease was responsible for over 750 thousand deaths, making it the leading cause of death for men over age 40. More people suffer from nervous and mental conditions in the twentieth century than in the last two centuries combined. In short, people are becoming sicker, waking up every morning to more bad news, with more confusion.

It is generally recognized that the United States is the most overmedicated, overoperated, overinoculated, and doctor-dependent country in the world. We have lost our self-reliance when it comes to health care and forgotten how to properly take care of ourselves. At the first sign of any symptom, we run to our doctor. If our doctor is not there to assist us or is unable to, we are left feeling hopeless and frustrated. Most people have no idea what to do when hit with a fever, taken down by a queasy stomach, or struck with a minor cough. This state of helplessness can really isolate and trap us. Our degree of dependence on the medical profession is pretty scary.

Furthermore, everybody wants a quick fix, something to make us feel healthier immediately. We want health the easy way, with no effort. When we lack energy, we want the energy pill; when we are overweight, we want the diet pill; when we are depressed, we want a pill to make us happy again. We tend to ignore the reasons why we have no energy or why we are overweight or depressed. We just want to be treated for it. Most people don't bother to contemplate that certain lifestyle choices may hold the answer, and making new choices may be all that is required of us.

With this in mind, you must try to become more active in your own health, without automatically running to the doctor to be fixed. And some people do think of themselves as a machine they can bring to their doctor's table with a request to be put back together—like a car or a television that needs repair.

You must understand which nutrients you need to make your body run, which foods keep you active and healthy rather than slow and sluggish, and how exercise can both stimulate you and relax you. After reading this book on clay as food and medicine, you will certainly have valuable information regarding many common health problems that will help you to avoid frequent trips to the doctor.

WE THOUGHT WE HAD DISEASES LICKED

Years ago, doctors thought diseases were a problem of the past. With the advent of antibiotics and penicillin, they felt they could control all the deadly microbes. But they claimed victory too soon. New scourges are emerging, and older diseases, like tuberculosis, are evolving into forms that antibiotics, the strongest weapon the doctor has, will no longer cure.

Germs have no boundaries. For all the massive power of modern medicine, deadly infections are a growing threat to everyone, everywhere. Here are some of the latest examples:

- 150,000 cases of a new form of hepatitis are occurring each year worldwide.
- Attacks of *E. coli* have ranged from Manhattan, where it found its way into the water supply, to the Pacific Northwest, where it hid in the hamburger meat of a well-known restaurant chain and killed three children.
- The hantavirus was identified in the Southwest, but not before 18 people died.
- Infections with streptococcus A, or the "flesh-eating bacteria," claim thousands of lives each year in the United States and Europe alone.
- Remember cholera? It's back—in a new, vaccine-immune strain. In Peru and Bolivia alone, a cholera epidemic made 740 thousand people ill in 1991 and

1992. In India, some infected adults have died in only nine hours.

- In 1993, more than 6,500 cases of whooping cough were reported nationwide, the highest incidence in more than 26 years.
- Lyme disease, another infectious disease, spreads quickly and is carried by tics. It has stricken at least 50,000 Americans since it was first discovered in 1976. The federal Centers for Disease Control and Prevention in Atlanta contend that many more people have been misdiagnosed.

The list goes on, but suffice it to say that it does not get any better. We are in serious trouble. Our allopathic (modern drug care) approach to disease has left us with our hands tied behind our backs. Newly emerging infectious diseases are a real and growing threat. Scientists say it's only a matter of time before another virus or new strain of bacterium attacks.

"We're vulnerable to something along the lines of the 1918–1919 influenza pandemic that killed 20 million people worldwide," says Dr. Robert Shope of Yale University. "It's happened once—it can happen again."

WHAT CAN WE DO?

We have viewed the problem of illness as something to attack and have used the metaphor "war on . . ." to describe the methods used. The metaphor is not limited, however, to medicine. We have a war on hate, a war on crime, a war on AIDS, and so on. I am not sure that looking at diseases from this perspective has helped us to solve them or even understand them better.

The natural view of disease is that health is dependent on balance and that we have become out of balance and must work to re-establish it. In health, the cells, tissues, and organs can survive only in delicate balance, made possible by the immune system. Once in harmony, they can effectively keep the body healthy and protect it from foreign invaders. Germs and microbes in themselves do not cause sickness. It's the immune system's vulnerability to germs and microbes that increases the risk for disease. When the immune system becomes strong, it may successfully protect itself against these vicious agents.

Perhaps "re-establish" is a better choice of words than "war on." Maybe we should talk about re-establishing peace, love, and health. Our language should imply working *with* rather than *against*. After all, what all natural medicine has in common is that it works with the subtle energies of the body and mind to create a better-functioning organism.

Our latest health policy waits for diseases to occur and then attempts to cut them off at the pass. For obvious reasons, this is no longer the safest or smartest way to approach illness. It is time to resort to a more intelligent medical system. I believe that natural medicine, with its emphasis on health prevention and maintenance rather than treatment of disease, offers a safe alternative.

THE NEW MILLENNIUM

Dr. Andrew Weil, author, professor, and medical doctor, best sums up the health-care industry in the new millennium in the title of his latest book: *Integrative Medicine*. We are witnessing the transformation of medicine and the eventual integration of conventional practice with naturopathic philosophies of care. Scientific research has been able to validate the old wisdom offered by natural medicine throughout the ages. This helps increase the effectiveness of diagnosis and cure and enhances our understanding of who we are as human beings in the modern world. The two branches of care are converging to create a stronger medicine—an integrative medicine.

Health care has been characterized by two distinct, separate philosophies of health: allopathy and naturopathy. These two philosophies have been like old, hardened cowboys, each wearing one-gallon hats, cowboy boots with spurs, and a holster with two guns. The cowboys lived in the same town but were always unwilling to share it with each other. They kept to their own business except to shoot at each other from time to time. "This hospital ain't big enough for the two of us," one of them would yell, pointing his gun at his nemesis' head and spitting on the ground. Allopathy and naturopathy were neighbors whom nobody thought would ever get along.

But things have changed since then. The cowboys are now sitting down with each other to have a drink in the saloon. On a good day, they play cards. However, these cowboys still have a long way to go.

This new type of thinking results in "integrative medicine," a system of health care that is concerned with the quality and preservation of life. At the time of this writing, in the United States, we are almost a quarter way toward a meeting of these divergent medical philosophies. Accredited naturopathic medical schools have found their way into our society and are asserting themselves as professional institutions. In the interest of gaining followers and establishing themselves as credible, they have developed a greater skill for diagnosis and a higher respect for available medical technology than their predecessors had. On the other side of the fence, elitist, conventional medical institutions such as Harvard and Yale have jumped on the "natural medicine" bandwagon. These schools offer an increased number of classes on various systems of naturopathic medicine for students interested in obtaining alternative perspectives on healing; this has come about in direct response to the popular demand for alternative means of care.

I believe that when people are ill, truly ill, all they really want is to feel better. They want to be cured. Whether that cure will come from a miracle drug or a two-thousand-year-old herb doesn't matter. They just want to feel good. When the two cowboys, allopathy and naturopathy, sit down for a drink and talk, they both recognize that.

"The people are gettin' onery," they say to one another. "They're sick and tired of us shootin' our guns and cavortin' in the streets. I'm willin' to put down these here pistols, pick up our medical books, and settle this feud once and for all. 'Cause if we don't, someone here may just get killed. And it may not be us—if you get what I mean." They nod at each other in solemn acknowledgment that if a patient dies this is the worst of all possible results.

Both these cowboys have something valuable to offer us. I hope for our sake and theirs that they put down their guns and pick up their medical books. People just want to get better in the new millenium.

WILL THE "NORMAL JOE SCHMOE" EVER EAT CLAY?

You may be wondering about all the excitement over natural medicine. Every time you turn on the television, it seems that a newscaster is talking about some "new and amazing" herb or natural substance. This week it may be an herb such as St. John's wort for depression, next week a shellfish derivative named glucosamine for arthritis, or two weeks from now the herb cat's claw for lack of energy. Why haven't you heard about eating clay more often? If herbs and other natural remedies are receiving national attention in the media, why hasn't eating clay become more popular with the mainstream by now?

Actually, in recent years it has been catching on. On March 19, 1997, the television show "Extra Magazine" broadcast a five-minute feature on eating clay—a major plug for geophagy, and some time ago (though I do not know the exact date) PBS aired an hour special on geophagy. A host of scientists, scientific experiments, conferences, and personal interviews offered an objective, informative view of this strange custom. I often run into articles in various newspapers and magazines that feature something about eating clay. I always smile when I see these new features on clay; they confirm my research that geophagy is a real and healthy practice.

But, I still wonder—if everyone in the world were absolutely convinced that eating clay was good for the body, and it could help them in the most extreme physical cases, would everyone take a bite?

The idea of eating dirt disgusts most people. Most civilized countries have become too "clean" and will not even think of eating dirt. People would sooner shower in chlorinated water, eat foods ridden with pesticides and herbicides, consume meats plugged up with synthetic hormones and antibiotics, and breathe cancerous fumes and vapors from factories, cars, and dyes than ever consider eating natural dirt from the earth! Never mind that the dirt will pull toxins from the body, stimulate the immune system, and absorb and bind pathogenic viruses, pesticides, and herbicides such as Paraquat and Roundup, in addition to many other functions. The thought of eating dirt sends shivers up some people's spines.

As for me, however, I'm not going to let a little grit between my teeth get in the way of health. I wrote this book to inform you of one of the earth's best-kept healing secrets. Clay has given many people a start on a new life. Let me emphasize from the very beginning that clay is not a miracle cure for disease, though I have witnessed miracle results in some people who have eaten clay. It is only one system of many natural therapies—but a wonderful one.

Everybody Eats Clay

A man may esteem himself happy when that which is his food is also his medicine.

Henry David Thoreau

There are many reasons why so many people of different ages, cultures, and races eat clay. Do these earth-eaters know something most people don't?

Yes, they do. Now you will know, too.

EIGHT REASONS FOR CLAY EATING

I have found eight basic reasons why people eat clay. They have more to do with survival and health than anything else.

1. Instinct
2. Medicinal uses
3. Detoxification
4. Mineral supplementation/deficiency
5. Religious rites
6. Famine food

7. Positive effects on pregnancy
8. A delicacy among certain cultures

Clay eating has nothing to do with climate, culture, race, or creed. It is found in the most "civilized" countries, where people like you or me do it, and among the most "primitive" tribes. The habit does not belong to any particular group, so no one can be clearly branded as clay-eaters and non-clay-eaters. In any one family, some persons will eat clay, and others will outright refuse. The habit is an individual one.

1. Instinct

Human beings have many inborn behaviors, or instincts. For instance, it is our very character to taste and test anything offered to us by nature; and eating clay, mud, or rocks is no more surprising than eating salt, herbs, chewing gum, tobacco, cows, or snails. These behaviors don't appear to be acquired through experience. Instead, they are most likely "in the genes" and are passed on from one generation to the next.

Children are the best examples of instinct. What child left in a sandbox will not grab a handful of dirt and shove it into his mouth? I don't know of many who won't. On the other hand, adults aren't as apt to play in a sandbox, so if their desire is for clay, they'll eat whatever they can get their hands on. According to Donald Vermeer, an anthropologist and a pioneer in the study of geophagy, many dirt-eaters in urban settings turn to the consumption of laundry starch or baking soda for want of clay. On a related note, many pregnant women feel the instinctual need to eat clay.

I believe that our bodies have an inborn knowledge of what is required to maintain health. When we react to these needs personally, on a gut level, we can find great healing. It is interesting that certain diseases such as dysentery (chronic diarrhea) or anemia predispose some of their sufferers to go out of their way to eat clay. For many persons, eating clay is as natural as the simple reflex actions of swallowing, breathing, and blinking.

2. Medicinal Uses

Clay eating has apparently been a recommended medicine for thousands of years, but most of us have not known about it, since such recommendations have been practically unheard of in the United States. Now that clay is becoming a more popular item in the health food stores, the word is getting around. Clay is said to do everything from acting as an intestinal evacuant and an alimentary detoxifier to working as a vermifuge (to get rid of parasites) and a natural antiviral and antibiotic.

If we go back through our history books, we'll see that Galen, the physician, introduced eating Armenian earth into medical practice to cure all sorts of ills, including acne and hemorrhoids. And a famous Taoist nicknamed Mud-pill Ch'en, known for his successful healing treatments with clay, cured diseases thought incurable in his time.

Incidentally, clay has always been touted as a cure for healing intestinal ailments. Mahatma Gandhi recommended earth to overcome constipation. And an institute in France uses clay in the manufacture of medicines to control and alleviate diarrhea in infants and adults.

But that's not all. On some islands in the South, the people have this cure for cholera: Leaves of an herb are placed in a jar of water with a ball of clay suspended above the preparation. The leaves are boiled, the ball of clay is crushed and stirred into the water, and this concoction is given to the patient to drink.

3. Detoxification

The *American Journal of Clinical Nutrition* published an article on clay eating and detoxification (Timothy and Duquette 1991). Among the many examples listed by the authors, the following are some of the more striking evidence for body purification through the use of clay. When the Pomo Indians of California consumed clay with traditionally bitter and toxic types of acorns, the clay adsorbed the poisons and eliminated the bitterness. The Indians were able to survive on a staple food that, without clay, would have posed a serious potential threat to their health.

In an experiment performed under laboratory conditions, rats voluntarily ate clay in response to gastrointestinal problems induced by poisoning. Further examples cited chimpanzees who ate clay after ingesting plant foods loaded with toxins.

The article concluded that clays could adsorb dietary toxins, bacterial toxins associated with gastrointestinal disturbance, hydrogen ions in acidosis, or metabolic toxins such as steroidal metabolites associated with pregnancy. All these conditions result in a host of common symptoms, including nausea, vomiting, and diarrhea—in short, symptoms of toxic overload.

4. Mineral Deficiency and Supplementation

Clay provides an impressive assortment of minerals, including calcium, iron, magnesium, potassium, sulfur, manganese, and silica as well as trace elements—those appearing in very tiny amounts. Without the basic minerals, life cannot exist; without the trace minerals, major deficiencies will develop. The lack of either will make it impossible for the body to maintain good health.

Most people don't realize the importance of minerals and

underestimate their legitimacy and use. This is too bad, because the body cannot manufacture its own minerals. Instead, they must be supplied by outside sources. Our need for minerals is as important as our need for air or water.

"The body can tolerate a deficiency of vitamins for a longer period of time than it can a deficiency of minerals. A slight change in the blood concentration of important minerals may rapidly endanger life," says F. P. Anita, M.D., in his book *Clinical Dietetics and Nutrition* (1989). Furthermore, mineral deficiencies can exacerbate symptoms caused by vitamin deficiency.

In most clays, the minerals exist in natural proportion to one another. This encourages their absorption by the intestinal tract. Accordingly, clay has been used by many tribes and cultures in the treatment of anemia and other mineral deficiencies.

5. Religious Rites

Many religions have made a positive connection between earth eating and spiritual and physical healing. Holy clay, the name for certain types of earth, is viewed as an extension of religious symbols through which transformation can take place.

In Esquipulas, Guatemala, home of the St. Esquipulas shrine, 5.7 million holy clay tablets are produced annually! The evolution of the Christian shrine here may have "Christianized" clay consumption. The tablet is seen as an extension of the power of the shrine and is believed to cure many illnesses, including ailments of the stomach, heart, eyes, and pelvis.

The tablets are prepared by hand, and pictures are carved on them. Two examples of the carvings include the crucifixion and resurrection. Stains of candy-makers' red dye are then daubed onto the tablets to represent the blood and wounds of Jesus. Interestingly, the Roman Catholic Church has indeed blessed medicinal clay tablets since the earliest days of Christianity, a millenium and a half before the statue of Esquipulas was carved.

Earth eating is also connected with religious belief among the Arabs and Muslims. In Mecca, clay is sold and stamped with the Arabic inscription "In the name of Allah! Dust of our land [mixed] with the saliva of some of us." It is thought that anyone who consumes this clay shares his or her spirit with Allah.

6. Famine Food

Grass, tree bark, wild herbs, weeds, and earth have always been primary food substitutes in famine times. With nothing left to eat, human beings will take whatever they can get their hands on—that is, anything to satisfy the stomach. Clay has been highly valued as a famine food because of its ability to calm hunger pangs. After eating clay, one feels full and, strangely, satisfied.

During a famine in China, one group sold what were called stone-cakes, which consisted of wood, pounded into dust and mixed with millet husks, then baked. It didn't look too bad, but it tasted like what it was—dust. Elsewhere, during the same famine, people made flour out of ground leaves, clay, and flower seeds. This was eaten as the daily diet until food could be found.

Different groups had many creative names for such food, calling it "mineral-flour," "earth-rice," or "stone-meal." Of course, in the end, it was really dirt they were eating. I suppose, however, it was better than chomping on boiled shoes, clothes, blankets, or leather.

7. Positive Effects on Pregnancy

Clay eating is most common during pregnancy. It is said to perform several functions, from supplying mineral nutrients to the unborn fetus to ensuring a safe delivery. But even when clay appears to make a dietary contribution, it is not eaten specifically for its nutrient content. The minerals may be viewed as a beneficial side effect.

In Malaysia, clay is eaten to help secure pregnancy by women who want to bear children. In New Guinea, pregnant women eat clay because they consider it good for the fetus. In Russia, one tribe considers clay placed on the tongue to be a good means of expediting birth and expelling the afterbirth. It is also taken to combat morning sickness.

People are quick to dismiss the earth cravings of pregnant women, since they often have desires for strange foods such as pickles and ice cream. But given the evidence from around the world, this practice doesn't seem so strange after all—just misunderstood.

8. A Delicacy among Cultures

Did you ever hear of eating chocolate-covered ants? As kids we used to joke about it. In India and Africa, however, this is no joking matter but a serious delicacy. People go to white ants' nests and eat the soil with the white ants included, sometimes adding honey to the preparation. They believe it's good for strength and energy.

While you and I would rather eat a piece of cake or a bowl of frozen yogurt, for many people clay with honey and sugar would be preferred. It sounds strange to us, but in cultures whose people have not been exposed to artificial flavors and colors, clay for dessert is a sure treat—and a healthy, low-calorie one at that.

Along the north coast of New Guinea, the people eat earth as a type of sweetmeat. The taste varies from faintly sweet to one very much like chocolate. Another group nearby takes pains to roll and form clay into disks and tubes, then cover the cakes with a solution of salt, smear them with coconut oil, and then roast and eat them.

EVEN ANIMALS EAT CLAY

Animals are instinctively drawn to clay, often when it is in the form of mud. I first read about animals eating clay in an article by Linda Clark, author of *Get Well Naturally,* who mentioned that elk, deer, coyote, and lynx gather in certain areas that contained clay. The animals lick the clay or, if injured, roll around in it to obtain relief from their injuries.

Later, I wasn't too surprised to learn how many other types of creatures also depend upon clay as an important part of their everyday diet:

- Brown and black bears eat clay in the late spring and summer in the Kenai peninsula of Alaska.
- Woodchucks, at times, are seen to eat gravel from roadsides.
- Butterflies are often observed to alight on moist soil surrounding puddles or on bars in streams. They ingest a little earth and then continue on their flight.
- Lambs in high-stocked areas who intuitively ate earth high in iodine, according to one field study, prevented the development of goiter.
- Rats eat clay in response to being poisoned.
- Many herbivorous animals will eat clay after ingesting herbs loaded with tannins, a toxic substance.

Certainly, animals are not exempt from clay eating. Yet, despite the numerous field studies and research reports, most scientists are unsure of the underlying reason or reasons why animals choose to ingest earth. I personally think it has something to do with health and that the animals are simply healthier for eating clay.

What Does Science Say about Clay?

Learn, compare, collect the facts!
Ivan Petrovich Pavlov

This chapter contains more scientific information than the rest of the book. However, the research available on eating clay is still very much in its beginning stages. If you understand the chemistry behind the clay, you can see how it works in the body. You'll know what therapeutic effects to look for and what hazards to watch out for. I promise to make everything here interesting and simple to read. As my dad says, "When I ask for the time, please tell me the time. And not how to build a clock."

TYPES OF CLAY

In a clay mineral the elements (oxygen, silicon, potassium, etc.) are spheres arranged in a regular three-dimensional pattern. The spheres are the building blocks of the clay minerals, and the arrangement of the spheres determines the type of mineral. The character of the clay mineral group determines

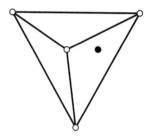

FIGURE 1. The three-dimensional pattern of the clay mineral. Whatever sits in the middle, in this case the silica element, determines the type of clay and what it will do. The name of this mineral structure is *single silica tetrahedron,* and it is the building block of montmorillonite clay (the best clay for eating).

the type of clay and its eventual use. In other words, the clay mineral structure gives us an understanding of its specific properties.

Among the clays suitable for eating, montmorillonite is the most common and most sought after. It has been the subject of many research studies and has long been recognized by scientists and laypersons for its unusual properties.

Montmorillonite clay was named after the town of Montmorillon, France, where it was first identified. The mineral clay belongs to a group of clays known as smectite, a word that describes its layered structure. The smectites are one of seven clay mineral groups. Each group contains a certain number of species, variations on the layered structure. Clay minerals come in many different shapes and sizes to produce a wide variety of clays.

Because there are so many types of clay, not all of them share the same function. Some are more suited for industrial use, whereas others are suited for dietary use. Of course, we are mainly interested in the clays that are best for internal use. However, before we begin to examine the different clay minerals, we must study two important properties that will help us define the minerals. As we do this, we will see why more value has been placed on certain clay minerals than on others.

ADSORB VERSUS ABSORB

Adsorption

The two words look alike, but their difference is critical in understanding the functions of clay minerals. *Adsorption* characterizes the process by which substances stick to the outside surface of the adsorbent medium. The clay possesses unsatisfied ionic bonds around the edges of its mineral particles. It naturally seeks to satisfy those bonds. For this to happen, it must meet with a substance carrying an opposite electrical (ionic) charge. When this occurs, the ions held around the outside structural units of the adsorbent medium and the substance are exchanged.

The particles of clay are said to carry a negative electrical charge, whereas impurities, or toxins, carry a positive electrical charge. For this very reason clay has been used to adsorb the colloidal impurities in beer, wine, and cider. The impurities in wine carry positive charges and can be coagulated (brought together) and removed by stirring a small amount of negatively charged clay material into the wine. The clay particles attract the wine impurities and they settle out together.

The process works the same in the human body. When clay is taken internally, the positively charged toxins are attracted by the negatively charged edges of the clay mineral. An exchange reaction occurs whereby the clay swaps its ions for those of the other substance. Now, electrically satisfied, it holds the toxin in suspension till the body can eliminate both.

The term *active*, or *alive*, indicates the ionic exchange capacities of a given clay mineral. The degree to which the clay-mineral ions become active determine its classification as alive. Living bodies are able to grow and change their form and size by taking within them lifeless material of certain kinds, and by transforming it into a part of themselves. No dead body can adsorb. It is physically impossible.

Absorption

Absorption is a much more slow and involved process than adsorption. Here, the clay acts more like a sponge, drawing substances into its internal structure. In order for absorption to occur, the substance must undergo a chemical change to penetrate the medium's barrier. Once it has done that, it enters between the unit layers of the structure. Instead of the toxins, for instance, sticking only to the surface, they are actually pulled inside the clay. This is the reason why absorptive clays are labeled expandable clays. The more substances the clay absorbs into its internal structure, the more it expands and its layers swell.

Any clay mineral with an inner layer charge is an absorbent. Having an inner layer charge means having charged ions, sitting between layers, that are surrounded by water molecules. In this way, the clay will expand as the substance to be absorbed fills the spaces between the stacked silicate layers.

A clay mineral with absorption properties can absorb virtually anything, whether it is a poison or soy sauce. As far as eating is concerned, however, you must make sure that your expandable clay minerals absorb only harmful toxins, not nutrients. Some clay minerals will absorb both and cause big problems by sucking in not only the poisons but the nutrients. If you are deficient in several nutrients that are necessary for health, you can easily become ill.

How exactly to know which clay is safe is really guess-work, unfortunately. Some clays are more gentle in their ab-sorption, whereas others are definitely more radical. Toward the end of the book, I will give you tips other people have given to me as well as those I have discovered myself for finding the right edible clay.

FIGURE 2.

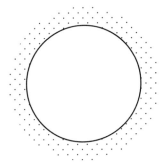

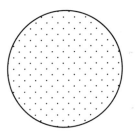

Adsorption: The tiny dots represent poisons; the large circle is the clay. Through ionic exchange, the harmful poisons are drawn to the out-side surface of the clay.

Absorption: The toxins have gone inside the clay and sit in between its layers.

WHICH CLAY WILL DO WHAT?

There are seven groups of clay. They are as follows:

Kaolin group
Illite group
Smectite group
Chlorite group
Vermiculite group
Mixed-layer group (consists of all five groups above)
Lath-form group

All clays will adsorb; however, the smectite group is the only one capable of absorption in addition to adsorption. Most clays sold in the health food industry belong to the smectite category. To save time and space, I will briefly review only the most popular clays.

Kaolin

Mentioned earlier, kaolin is the mineral clay used in Kaopectate. While it adsorbs toxins and bacteria like the other clays, it primarily acts as a bulking agent and serves an antidiarrheal purpose. Recently, several health food companies have advertised kaolin as a part of their mineral complexes, emphasizing its trace mineral benefits.

Illite

The illite group is named for the state of Illinois. The best-known species of illite is glauconite, a green mineral clay. It is typically found in clays of marine origin. Other colors include white and yellow.

Smectite

Smectite is characterized by its expandable properties. Unlike the other clays, only smectite can absorb as well as adsorb toxins. This qualifies its structural uniqueness and sets it apart from all other clays. For this reason, smectite has become a favorite clay for industrial and dietary use.

The most familiar species of smectite is montmorillonite. Again, it is the most preferred species of edible clay, next to green clay. Most research has been done with montmorillonite.

What Makes Montmorillonite So Special?

The montmorillonite minerals occur in very small particles. They are extremely fine-grained and thin-layered, more so than any of the other clay minerals. The layers contain ions that are very loosely bound to one another and easily exchangeable. Not only will the toxins stick to its outside surface, but numerous elements and organic matter will enter the space between the layers.

In addition to its already unique structure, montmorillonite has a particularly large surface area when properly hydrated in water, which further boosts its adsorptive and absorptive properties. Chemically and structurally, it is shaped like a credit card, with negative charges on the flat surface and positive charges at the edges. Therefore, the negative charge (the good one) is many times more poweful than the positive charge. Montmorillonite is a more complicated clay and has a higher exchange capacity then the simpler species of clay, such as kaolinite. Its ability to adsorb and absorb toxins is greater than that of the clays in the other groups.

According to one article on clay (Lei 1996), a mineralogist at Massachussetts Institute of Technology, Robert T. Marin, stated that one gram of this clay has a surface area of 800 square meters. To give that some serious perspective, that's about ten football fields! The greater the surface area of the clay, the greater the power to pick up positively charged particles or toxins many times its own weight.

Any given clay is usually a mixture of clay minerals, one or two minerals almost always being predominant. Clays are rarely found separately and are usually mixed not only with other clays but with microscopic crystals of quartz, mica, feldspar, and carbonates. Most clay contains montmorillonite to a greater or lesser degree. The available types of montmorillonite vary in color, consistency, and shape. The color may be white, gray, or pink, with tints of yellow or green. Typically, montmorillonite will be included in a mixture of clay groups in any given material; all six clay groups will most likely contain particles of montmorillonite. Sources of montmorillonite include the United States, Italy, and France.

Bentonite

You may have heard of bentonite, a much-used industrial clay. Currently, several companies are selling bentonite in their health formulas. Bentonite is widely distributed in nature. Its name was derived from the Fort Benton series of cretaceous rocks in Wyoming, where it was first found. The name can be misleading; bentonite is not a mineral name but a trade name for a commercially sold swelling clay. It is often used in commerce as a name for montmorillonite, and sometimes the names are used interchangeably. Smectite is the general group name used by mineralogists.

The source of bentonite is weathered volcanic ash. In marine environments, the ash transforms itself, over time, to smectite. There are several species in the smectite group, montmorillonite being one of them. Depending on its source, bentonite may contain a high percentage of montmorillonite or just a tiny bit. The rest of the contents may either be related or a completely different mineral group. Rarely will you ever find a 100 percent pure smectite; therefore, not all bentonite is a pure smectite. Quite commonly, the clay minerals illite or chlorite are present in alternating layers.

When we choose and eat the right clay, we need to be aware of this. Bentonite is sometimes wrongly sold under the montmorillonite label or, at least, the name doesn't give any clear indication of its contents. I have seen a wide variety of bentonite clays where each one looked, felt, tasted, and acted differently from the others. They did so because they were not the same clays. The variation in minerals does not really matter in industrial use, so long as the bentonite has good expansion capacity. But the guidelines for industry use do not hold for the consumption of clay. Unfortunately, because some clays vary in contents, some are better suited than others for eating.

This tends to be confusing, and it seems uncertain exactly which clay mineral you are getting even when the label tells you "bentonite." Even the scientists have differing opinions or are not sure themselves.

Single- and Mixed-Clay Minerals

Typically, any given clay material may be composed of particles of a single clay mineral or a complex of many different naturally occurring minerals. It is not easy to find pure samples of many of the clay minerals. When they are found in nature, like a vein of gold, they are painstakingly mined. Otherwise, scientists depend on preparing single-clay minerals in the laboratory.

Most commonly in nature, layers of one type—for example,

montmorillonite—are interlayered with units of another type, for example, illite. In other words, a tiny particle may be composed of successive layers of illite and montmorillonite. This of course varies according to the region of the deposit and the climate. Climactic effects influence the occurence of certain clay minerals.

SUMMARY

The actions of any clay material are difficult to predict because of this complicated makeup. Unfortunately, there is no simple relationship between the chemical components of the clay minerals and their actions. While some clay minerals will look almost identically alike, their actions will differ radically. By the same token, though certain clay minerals structurally share nothing in common, their actions may mimic each other.

The fact is that nobody in the geophagy or geochemistry world knows everything there is to know about clay. At best, the information is sporadic and limited. I have indeed only touched the tip of the iceberg.

If this leaves you unsure and nervous about eating clay, you can investigate the different clay minerals. There is an infinite number of clay minerals to be researched, but I'm not so sure that research is very important. All you really need to be familiar with are the main mineral groups so you can see patterns emerging in relation to therapeutic effects.

In chapter 10 I include more information on purchasing the right clay for your needs. And throughout the book I give you simple guidelines for choosing the right clay. Do not worry about picking up a jar of clay off the shelves of a health food store and eating something dangerous, or not getting what you paid for. Most companies in the industry are committed to supplying the best product and have no desire to cheat the consumer. They are interested in selling their wares, and they hope you will return to buy more. Further, health food stores will do their best to stock the highest-quality product, especially one that poses no risk (of any kind) to themselves or the consumer. Thus, edible clays you find in the health food store generally should be safe for consumption.

Clay Is Alive

*Viewed from the distance of the moon, the aston-
ishing thing about the earth . . . is that it is alive.*

Lewis Thomas, *Lives of a Cell:
Notes of a Biology Watcher*

The universe is made up of living and nonliving systems. Most
people agree on what is alive in this world. The human body,
for example, is a living system. It is made up of a group of
working cells, which develop into organs like the heart or
lungs to support the body in its functions: to grow, reproduce,
and support life. Plant life, like the body, follows a similar
pattern and therefore belongs to the living system. Plants follow the pattern of living, reproducing, and growing, giving
witness to the cycle of life and death.

Rocks, on the other hand, are incapable of growing and
reproducing. They fall into the category of nonliving systems.
They are inert. A rock will do only one thing: decompose, or
fall apart into simpler and simpler elements. The only way a
rock will structurally change is through the weathering process, for instance, whereby the elements control its change. On
its own, it can do nothing.

Only when a living organism dies does it become subject

to the laws of the nonliving world, falling away into simpler and simpler components. The difference beween a living organism and one newly dead is that "something" we call life, which we can neither see, hear, smell, touch, nor weigh, but which animates the physical body while it is still alive. This force has the power to counteract disintegration and decay (Gibson and Gibson 1987).

In basic science class we learn that the building blocks of matter are atoms. The last 20 years of research and study, however, have shown us these atoms are more complex than was originally thought, and break down into tinier, subatomic particles. These particles carry either a positive or a negative electrical charge; some are neutral, and others appear as if they have no weight. It is the combination and arrangement of these particles that form simple, inorganic elements like salt and water and more complex organic substances elaborated by living systems.

Yet, behind this awesome spectacle of nature, these particles alone are insufficient to generate life. A particle by itself can do nothing without the life force animating its being. This animating principle is the "something" that organizes and directs the entire process.

THE ONE-MILLION-YEAR EXPERIMENT

If you were to place a couple of tablespoons of clay in a jar of water and return one million years later, you would find that the clay you would come back to is not the same one you had left behind. It changed to another mineral.

That's because the chemical and physical components in the clay are constantly shifting. The clay is alive. According to Dr. Don Burt, professor of geology at Arizona State University, certain clays are unstable and will restructure themselves over time. For example, under certain conditions volcanic ash will turn to smectite. And smectite, in turn, will change to kaolinite, certain conditions permitting. Thus, the elements are kept in continous motion, charged by an unseen life force. This is the definition of an active clay mineral. Being active, it changes, grows, and reconfigures itself.

ENERGY EXCHANGE

If we go back to our base physical components, we can safely say that we are built from multitudes of particles held together by electrical bonds. Electrical forces are what hold atoms and molecules together. Chemical bonds and reactions depend on these electrical forces. Therefore, all chemical reactions are, in essence, reorganizations of electrical forces, which continue to be vital at body levels, i.e., tissues and organs. When this is all taken into account, a living organism is shown to be an extremely intricate electrical system (Gibson and Gibson 1987).

During illness, the vital force is weak and incapable of supporting the body and its functions. In health, however, the opposite occurs: the force is strong and is able to counteract sickness and decay. What keeps the immune system running is the energy that feeds it, the substance of life. The body will not run well, or will at least run with all sorts of mechanical problems, when there is no energy to support it.

When clay is consumed, its vital force is released into the physical body and mingles with the vital energy of the body, creating a stronger, more powerful energy in the host. Its particles are agents of stimulation and transformation capable of withholding and releasing energy at impulse. The natural magnetic action transmits a remarkable power to the organism and helps to rebuild vital potential through the liberation of latent energy. When it is in contact with the body, its very nature compels it to release its vital force: the same vital force from which so many plants and animals feed.

Therefore, in order to create health, the body must be stimulated and restimulated by another working energy like clay. When the immune system does not function at its best, the clay stimulates the body's inner resources to awaken the stagnant energy. It supplies the body with the available magnetism to run well.

Does that mean you have to be sick to take clay? No, not at all. The best-known characteristic of clay is that it "acts as needed." Clay is said to propel the immune system to find a new healthy balance. Reactions are not forced, but rather triggered into effect as they are needed. To put it into other words, clay simply strengthens the body to a point of higher resistance. In this way, the body's natural immune system has an improved chance of restoring and maintaining health.

Clay Interacting with Life

The doctor of the future will give no medicine but will interest his patients in the care of the human frame in diet and in cause and prevention of disease.

Thomas A. Edison

This chapter gives a brief overview of clay and mineral supplementation. It may therefore seem out of place with the rest of the book, which focuses on clay's unique ability to draw toxins out of the body because it is not absorbed itself. It seems entirely paradoxical that clay can function both as a detoxifier and as a source of substances the body can absorb. Logic would tell us that there is no means by which clay could act as an inert substance in one moment, and in the next function as a substance capable of fulfilling nutritional needs. It is like taking a circular block and placing it into a square hole and succeeding! But it is true: clay has the capacity to function as both.

Since much more research is needed to give a better understanding of clay and how it works, namely, an explanation of this paradox, this chapter will not be able to shed light on this problem. It will, however, examine one aspect of clay eating that is sometimes not well reported: that clay can be a beneficial source of minerals. Supplementation with minerals has received a lot of attention in the media lately. Because certain varieties of clay contain minerals in nutritionally significant amounts, it can successfully be taken as a dietary supplement.

A SOURCE OF NUTRIENTS

According to an article published in the *American Journal of Clinical Nutrition,* "Detoxification and Mineral Supplemenation As Functions of Geophagy" (Johns and Duquette 1991), the most prevalent explanation of clay eating is that it is a response to nutritional deficiency. In several clinical studies, eating clay has been implicated as a *response* to particular deficiencies. But there are many studies that implicate it as a *cause* of particular deficiencies, too.

In a handful of experiments run by scientists, mineral deficiencies, such as those for iron or potassium, were introduced to animals. As a result of those experiments, those animals changed in their dietary behavior. For instance, iron deficiency has been established as a reason for the ingestion of certain clays, although there is still debate on this issue. In the Runjut Valley, in the Sikkim Himalayas, the natives chew a red clay as a cure for goiter because of its particular mineral content. It is not uncommon for mineral supplements in health food stores to contain portions of various types of clay. Certain clays, though not all clays, contribute major amounts of important minerals, such as calcium, iron, magnesium, manganese, and zinc.

MINERALS AND CLAY

Minerals are present in living tissue and are essential to all chemical reactions in the body. However, the body cannot manufacture its own minerals, and they must therefore be supplied by an outside source. Without minerals, the body will easily succumb to disease.

What Do Minerals Do?

Minerals perform a number of important functions. They:

1. Supply major elements and trace elements that may be lacking in the diet.
2. Act as catalysts, thus playing a major role in metabolism and cell building.
3. Regulate the permeability of cell membranes.
4. Maintain water balance and osmotic pressure between the inside and outside environment.
5. Influence the contractility of muscles.
6. Regulate the response of nerves to stimuli.

Why are minerals so important to the chemical reactions in the human body? The cell is like an electrical battery with positive and negative charges. When the energy of the battery begins to weaken, the cell becomes sick and weak. However, if the dying cell is charged by an electrical current, it will become living once again. Minerals themselves hold positive and electrical charges. The exchange of these charges accounts for its action. Scientists are not sure exactly how this works or to what degree it does. Yet, when we give the cell the essential minerals it needs to live, it can regenerate and "nurse" itself back to health.

What would happen if your body lacked the essential minerals it needs? Here are some minerals and the beneficial role they play:

Calcium: essential to the formation of strong bones and teeth.

Iodine: keeps the thyroid gland running.

Iron: vital to the blood, carries oxygen; a lack of it can cause anemia.

Magnesium: necessary to food metabolism and nerve function.

Phosphorus: regulates heart, nerve, and muscle activity and helps to maintain acid–alkali balance in the blood and tissues.

Potassium: plays a role in maintaining water and pH balance in addition to strengthening the nerves and heart.

Selenium: once thought to be toxic, today recognized as one of the most valuable elements; it works as an antioxidant, a major factor in the prevention of cancer.

Sodium: helps regulate water and pH balance; too much can cause edema, swelling of the tissues.

Zinc: important to the functions of the eyes and, in men, a working prostate.

Today, we know the functions of most major minerals, such as the ones listed above. Yet, we still do not understand the role of the more obscure minerals, such as gold or tin. In the future, I am sure we will discover their purpose. As we learn more about the effects of increasing human health through mineral supplementation, their value will be emphasized.

What Quantity of Minerals Do You Need to Stay Healthy?

Mineral elements enter into the structure of every cell of the body. Certain structures contain more elements than others, each according to its specific need. For instance, bones contain more calcium and magnesium than soft tissues, which contain, for instance, more phosphorus.

There are no traditional data on the amount of trace elements necessary for human function. Minerals at one time thought to be toxic, such as selenium and chromium, have been found to be essential to many chemical reactions in the body. Selenium, for instance, is recognized for its cancer-fighting properties, whereas chromium is needed as an essential element in controlling metabolism and blood sugar levels.

Exactly how much of each mineral is needed, however, no one can determine. A small amount of an element does not give any indication of our need for it and bears no relationship to its importance. We know the pivotal role calcium plays and that without a 1000-mg daily dose our bones might become brittle and our nerves weak and jittery. But who would have ever thought about the trace element cobalt, whose 5 mg per day is absolutely vital in the form of vitamin B_{12}? Too little cobalt would result in a serious drop in physical energy.

Proportion is a key factor in the proper assimilation of minerals by the body. Scientific understanding cannot account for the role minerals play in combination with each other. A shortage of one mineral can have a harmful influence on the role of another and, in turn, change the requirement for still another. For instance, an excess of zinc can lead to a copper deficiency, or too much calcium can ruin your magnesium uptake. Persons must be very careful when dosing themselves with various mineral supplements. There are immediate dangers.

A Sample of Clay

Exactly how many minerals does the typical clay compound contain? One analysis of a montmorillonite clay found in Nevada contains the following elements:

Aluminum	Holmium	Ruthenium
Antimony	Indium	Samarium
Arsenic	Iodine	Scandium
Barium	Iridium	Selenium
Beryllium	Iron	Silicon
Bismuth	Lanthanum	Silver
Boron	Lead	Sodium
Bromine	Lithium	Strontium
Cadmium	Lutecium	Sulfur
Calcium	Magnesium	Tantalum
Cerium	Manganese	Tellurium
Cesium	Mercury	Terbium
Chlorine	Molybdenum	Thallium
Chromium	Neodymium	Thorium
Cobalt	Nickel	Thulium
Copper	Niobium	Tin
Dysprosium	Osmium	Titanium
Erbium	Palladium	Tungsten
Europium	Phosphorus	Uranium
Fluorine	Platinum	Vanadium
Gadolinium	Potassium	Ytterbium
Gallium	Praseodymium	Yttrium
Germanium	Rhenium	Zinc
Gold	Rhodium	Zirconium
Hafnium	Rubidium	

You may be surprised at the amount of elements present in a clay mineral sample. Indeed, it is astounding. Yet, believe it or not, most people who eat the clay do not eat it for its mineral content. Instead, they view that part as an added benefit.

Unfortunately, I was unable to receive from this company an analysis of the exact mineral percentages contained in the clay sample. It is important to obtain an analysis of mineral composition in order to verify there is not a high percentage of certain toxic minerals. Since variation among clays can occur, individuals should request such an analysis when they purchase clay. However, if an analysis is not immediately available, this may not be cause for worry. It is common practice for any company selling clay for ingestion to perform a mineral analysis. As a matter of fact, it is a practical safeguard that is expected of that company. Most companies that supply health food stores are voluntarily regulated by a national independent foods association, in the interest of attracting consumers, and they adhere to strict quality standards. No one wants to be sued.

I'll Take Minerals, But Not *Those* Minerals!

In looking for the right clay, the objective is to locate a particular clay whose mineral content is suitable for digestion. The fact that elements exist inside the clay in an organic form does not ensure that they are safe for eating. One does not want to eat a clay loaded with the minerals arsenic or cadmium, for instance. That would be close to suicide, since these minerals are highly toxic.

Ideally, nobody wants a clay containing toxic minerals. So, what happens if your clay has naturally occurring amounts of arsenic or cadmium? Does this pose a problem if you would like to eat clay? The answer is "no." Or, at least, "no, so long as the minerals are present in trace amounts." That may sound strange, but read on. In the absorption of toxic metals, a hierarchy is involved. First, in order for minerals to be absorbed they must bind to an enzyme. Second, both toxic and nontoxic minerals bind to the same enzymes. Third, when there are large amounts of major nontoxic elements and microtrace amounts of toxic elements, they compete to bind on the same enzyme. As a result, the toxic elements are essentially "outnumbered" and therefore cannot be absorbed very readily. Granted, the undesired toxic elements will bind much more strongly to the enzyme, but if there is a good supply of nontoxic metals, then the former are not absorbed properly.

Since I have already mentioned the presence of cadmium in clay, let me give an example involving this mineral and the hierarchical nature of toxic metal absorption. Even though clay may contain cadmium, if 200 times as much zinc and copper are present, the cadmium will not be absorbed. If however, there exists a significant lack of zinc and copper, then it would not be in the individual's best interest to eat the clay—the toxic mineral cadmium would be well absorbed. In the end, eating clay with a tiny percentage of toxic metals may feel a bit strange, but the information available here concerning toxic metal absorption is well documented and is fundamental to toxicology.

Minerals and Our Food Supply

Since the advent of chemical fertilizers, herbicides, pesticides, and fungicides, the soil our vegetables and fruits grow in has been virtually depleted of its vital trace elements. These elements, minute in quantity, determine the nutritional value of what we eat.

A boron deficiency in apples results in a wrinkled and weathered-looking fruit. A magnesium deficiency in grapefruit results in a deterioration of its leaves—but that's just what you see on the outside.

Currently, in an attempt to make up for this lack of minerals, many farmers must supply their soil with magnesium, boron, manganese, copper, and/or zinc. But this doesn't take care of the problem. For instance, a soil low in iron may be sprayed with additional iron. But that same soil may still be iron deficient if it contains toxic amounts of copper or zinc. The point is that poor soil leads to poor quality of food. And a diet lacking in nutrients leads to an unhealthy body. This is why clay may be such a valuable source of the major and trace elements.

Moustached Tamarins

In an experiment set up to discover some of the reasons why primates eat clay, scientists reached the conclusion that they were fulfilling their mineral needs. The scientists set up a field study at the Rio Blanco in northeastern Peru from June to September, where they observed moustached tamarins, primates in the Amazon, feeding on soil material.

They noted that these primates would eat soil only from ant nests, not the plain old dirt on the ground. When the scientists wondered why these primates preferred one particular soil to all others, they made their amazing discovery. An analysis of the soil from the broken mound of leaf-cutting ants revealed that the concentration of several elements was much higher. The soil material used by ants stems from deeper soil layers which are less leached than the surface soil.

The months July to September receive, on average, less rain than the other months and also represent a period of relative fruit scarcity. The overall mineral uptake of the moustached tamarins is reduced during this period. This further explains why the primates preferred one particular soil over others at this time.

The question of taste never entered into the scientists' conclusion. Taste never had any bearing on the primates' choices. No special taste was apparent among any of the samples, except that one of the samples had a very light salty taste—and the threshold for salty taste is even lower in moustached tamarins than in humans.

In the end, the most likely functional explanation for why these primates eat clay is mineral supplementation. Some of the more interesting facts included in the article were other reasons why primates, other than moustached tamarins, eat clay. They include absorption of plant toxins, adjustment of pH in the stomach, and tactile sensation in the mouth.

In the past, little emphasis has been placed on the role minerals play in nutrition. Now, this has changed. The importance of meeting nutritional mineral requirements can no longer be doubted.

AMINO ACIDS AND CLAY

Amino acids are the building blocks of life that make up proteins, which are essential to life. They are a primary ingredient of most cell structures. Proteins are essential to all the chemical processes of the cells and thus are needed to rebuild the constant wear and tear on the human body. For instance, high-protein diets are especially vital during the growth years, during pregnancy, and when tissue has been damaged by injury or disease.

Some research has shown that certain clays may have played an essential role in the formation of life. This hypothesis comes from experiments performed with clay to recreate the conditions under which amino acids may form proteins. In the laboratory, tests showed that single amino acids formed into the longer chains called peptides on the surface of clay particles. The clay is thought to act as a pattern and catalyst for the formation of long peptide chains, or proteins. Scientists added a small amount of one amino acid to a solution of various clay minerals. They then exposed the clay to varying degrees of temperature and moisture. The main findings were that more peptides were produced at various temperatures when clay was present than when it was absent, and that the production of peptides was higher in the presence of the changes in temperature and moisture. Protein conversion can sometimes fail to proceed normally through the peptide chains in the human body and, as a result, prevent their use.

On the basis of these findings, published in *Scientific American* (Millot 1979), the investigators proposed that the fluctuation of temperature and moisture brings about a distribution and redistribution of amino acids on the surface of clay particles that favors the amino acids' linkage into peptide chains. When moisture touches the surface of the clay mineral, the active sites on the surface that speed the formation of peptides are cleaned. Then, when the same water used to clean the surface evaporates because of the change in temperature, new catalytic sites become available for other amino acids to form new chains. This ongoing cycle, totally dependent upon the clay minerals, is synonymous with life.

Tell Me More about Clay

If purpose, then, is inherent in art, so is it in Nature also. The best illustration is the case of a man being his own physician, for Nature is like that—agent and patient at once.

Aristotle, *Physics*

HEALING THE NATURAL WAY

One of the great advantages to eating clay is that there are no contraindications for its use. One doesn't have to worry about existing conditions such as high blood pressure, diabetes, allergies, hormone imbalances, or high triglyercides or cholesterol levels when eating clay on a daily basis. Clay has never been known to have an adverse effect on any of these chronic ailments. Unlike certain natural substances, such as the herb ma huang, which are not advisable because of existing health conditions that make their use dangerous, clay is safe for consumption. Users may reap the positive benefits of eating it without worrying about harmful side effects.

As a safe addition to the diet, clay is an easily recommendable item. The worst situation that could befall any person who begins to eat clay would be that he or she fails to see any results. If this happens, then no real harm has been done. But in most cases, clay-eaters see great effects and continue eating the clay for quite some time.

There are clays, as already mentioned in chapter 3, that you will want to avoid, however. Some clays are not meant to be eaten. Again, there is no real need to worry about this if you're purchasing your clay at a health food store. There are some really excellent brands on the shelves today. On the other hand, if you decide to travel to foreign countries and eat the dirt in obscure places, talk to the local residents before you make a possibly bad mistake!

Clay can be taken to charge the immune system during an ongoing disease, and it can also be taken as a preventive, to help ward off any potential ailments. Ideally, clay should be taken to build immunity, so that if you are exposed to a contagious illness or if you are approaching a time of lowered resistance, your defense system is prepared. This all boils down to one thing: if we want to keep healthy we need to keep our immune system functioning at its best. Clay contains the minerals and energy that the defense mechanism needs; it improves bowel function and detoxifies the body of pollutants. So, it makes sense that one of the best ways to stay healthy and keep disease away is to eat clay.

THE BASIC CAUSE OF DISEASE

Health depends on three factors:

1. Eating good, nourishing foods.
2. Absorbing those foods properly so your cells don't starve.
3. Eliminating all the waste matter from your system.

First, to live vibrantly, the foods that feed the body must be the right kind—that is, they must contain the vitamins, minerals, and enzymes necessary to feed the cells. Hippocrates was correct when he said, "Your food shall be your medicine and your medicine shall be your food." Whatever we put into the body is automatically used for its growth, maintenance, and repair. That is exactly how food acts as medicine. A balanced diet provides the building blocks of a healthy body.

Second, the body must properly assimilate the foods to receive their vital nutrients. When the food enters the small intestine, the pancreas and small bowel wall must send juices and bile to individually digest the carbohydrates, proteins, and fat. That's a lot of work for a healthy system, much more so for one that is already sick. If the body cannot perform this job, then the cells become weakened and starve.

Third and last is the importance of elimination. For many years people in the natural health field have told us that poor bowel health causes and aggravates disease conditions. Now, research is beginning to substantiate these beliefs. John Tilden, M.D., author of *Toxemia* (1974), states that the basic cause of disease is insufficient drainage of waste matter: that toxins have accumulated in the blood above the toleration point, and disease—call it a cold, a flu, a headache—is the result of an accumulation of poisons in the system.

If the system fails to get rid of poisons through the bowels, a constipated condition arises in which the toxins never leave the body. They sit inside and putrefy. What's worse, the body doesn't know the difference between live food and dead food in the colon. It will still try to get nourishment out of waste you would never want to set your eyes upon. Naturally, this puts a strain on every functioning cell in the body.

THE CLAY AT WORK

The clay's immediate action upon the body is directly on the digestive channel. This involves the clay actually binding with the toxic substances and removing them from the body with the stool. It performs this job with every kind of toxin, including those from the environment, such as heavy metals, and those that occur naturally as by-products of the body's own health processes, such as metabolic toxins. It's hard to believe that the body produces its own toxins, but that may happen as a result of stress, inefficient metabolism, or the proliferation of free radicals.

The body has no problem ridding itself of the clay. Don't worry about a tiny brick house being built in the middle of your colon. The clay assists the body's eliminatory process by acting as a bulking agent, similar to psyllium fiber, sweeping out the old matter that doesn't need to be there. It is not digested in the same manner as food as it passes through the alimentary canal. Instead, it stimulates intestinal peristalsis, the muscular contractions that move food and stool through the bowels. The clay and the adsorbed toxins are both eliminated together; this keeps the toxins from being reabsorbed into the bloodstream.

ODE TO VITAMINS

A commonly asked question is whether or not clay will destroy vitamins. In other words, can it resist sucking up the "good stuff" in the intestinal tract while it sucks up all the "bad stuff"? Unfortunately, there is no straight answer to this question; that really depends on the mineral clay being ingested. Because all clays vary in their consistency, taste, and color, their actions will differ. Some will enhance or expand the potency of whatever supplements you take, while others will steal the nutrients for all they are worth.

Most clays sold for consumption in the health food stores are okay to eat. Unlike potentially harmful clays, which may absorb everything, these clays should pose no serious health risk. Furthermore, these clays have typically been analyzed for their mineral components, and in this case you will know what you are getting.

However, beware of any clays whose labels tell you to load up on a wide array of vitamins after you take them. If this is the program they call for, the clay's absorbing power goes far beyond that of absorbing toxins. In all probability, this clay is not safe for regular consumption. Healthy persons may use these types of clays once in a while when nothing better is available, but they should never make a regular habit of it. Young children, pregnant women, and persons with low vitality, however, should stay away from these types of mineral clays. When vital energy is needed the most, they will cause the body to work harder than normal. Taken on a daily basis, they will weaken the cells, sap the body of strength, ruin elimination, and finally lead to the very thing the body tries to desperately avoid: disease.

The ideal clay is one that will adsorb and absorb the poisons, as well as enhance or expand whatever nutrients you put into your body. For instance, if you take the herbs ginseng and garlic, or the antioxidant pycnogenol, you should benefit from greater assimilation because of the clay's action as an intestinal cleanser and gastrointestinal regulator. As the body cleans house, it is in a better position to more efficiently assimilate the much-needed nutrients.

Unfortunately, many people take a handful of supplements but never reap the desired effects because of a malfunctioning colon. Whereas a healthy person will digest most of whatever food substance he or she puts into the body, someone whose colon function is deficient may digest very little. Although new health programs may be introduced, sometimes the person is still left feeling run-down, cranky, and sick. Clay can be an important part of one's health program because it assists colon function. Then, whatever supplements are taken in addition to the clay will be better used by the body because the body will have the means to do so.

CLAY AND MEDICATION

Clay should not be eaten within three hours before or after having taken medication because it will interfere with effective natural digestion of most drugs. ("Medication" here refers to any sort of drug, not a supplement.)

Unfortunately, very little scientific research on clay's interaction with drugs is available. But, when rats ate clay after being poisoned, repeated doses of clay prevented gastrointestinal absorption of the poison, which continued for up to 30 hours. This supports the opinion of many physicians, both alternative and allopathic, that clay and medication should not be taken at the same time. Because of clay's absorptive and adsorptive abilities, it draws synthetic medicines into its sphere and renders them ineffective to protect the body. This is not a useful result if one relies on medication.

All this does not mean, however, that one cannot eat clay if taking medicine. It simply means that adjustments to medication and clay-eating schedules must be made such that neither will have any specific influence on the other. Also, take no more than one or two doses of clay per day.

Before changing any prescribed medications, consult your physician.

Note to the elderly: Avoid clay for three to five hours after taking medication.

EXPECT A DIFFERENCE

If you have never eaten clay before and plan on eating it for the first time, expect a real treat! Even though we seem to know quite a bit about the clay, how it works, and what it does, its true actions still remain a mystery. Here are what most people have to say about clay eating after only two to four weeks of use:

- Well-regulated bowels.
- Relief from constipation or diarrhea.
- No more indigestion.
- No more ulcers.
- Better digestion of food and drink.
- A surge in physical energy.
- Less "wandering pain" all over the body.
- Clearer skin.
- Whiter and brighter eyes.
- More alertness and clear-headedness.
- Emotional uplift, less tension.
- Enhanced growth and tissue repair of gums and skin.
- Stimulated the immune system, higher resistance to infectious agents.

As you can see, clay works on the entire organism. No one part of the body is left untouched by its healing energies. I don't know of another supplement that is quite as capable as clay of producing such a wide range of positive reactions.

The effects of clay are wide and varied, and I am always amazed at new cures that result when persons eat dirt. For example, someone takes clay for energy and winds up with improved eyesight. Another person eats clay to assimilate food better and ends up having more energy. All reported benefits are common results of increasing digestive and eliminatory efficiency. It's absolutely weird and wonderful. In the end, I have no reasonable explanation for why the clay works in this curious fashion.

I'LL EAT CLAY FOR A LONG TIME

Clay works best when taken over a long period of time. That's because its actions are subtle. Like a snowball rolling down the hill, it starts off small and slow. As it continues to roll, it soon picks up momentum and goes faster. Clay does not offer instant cures for all ailments, but history shows it can encourage the body to put up a better fight when taken over a long period of time.

When clay is taken for indefinite periods of time, it has no addictive qualities. This is a big concern for many who begin eating the clay. The effects can be so positive that it scares them into thinking they might need it forever. However, one can quit eating clay at any time. There are no withdrawal symptoms, and you will never need to enter a withdrawal program.

Many people ask me, on the other hand, if the clay is something they have to take for the rest of their life. The answer to the question, of course, is they don't have to; there is no risk in discontinuing its use. But, why not take something that is good for you and will help to clean out your body? Especially in today's highly polluted world, our liver and kidneys are so overworked they never have a chance to rest. Personally, I want to help out my kidneys and liver by making their job easier. And if taking a spoonful of dirt every day helps them to work better and keeps my mind and body functioning in tip-top condition, I'll eat clay for a long time.

DRINK LOTS OF WATER

It is said that the average person should drink between six and eight glasses of water per day. This rule is especially important to a person who eats clay. Clay needs water to perform its job. Like a sponge, it cannot absorb anything if it is dry. You must drink lots of water if you want to get the best results from the clay treatment.

The more water you drink, the better the clay will work. Try this simple test at home. Put some clay powder into a bowl, then drop a couple of teaspoons of water into the bowl. Watch how the clay immediately sucks the water into its internal structure. That's exactly what happens in the body. But if the clay doesn't have water to work with, it can't do its job, or will not do it well.

If the clay can't do its job, you won't see any effects. The clay will be eaten every day, but nothing good will come of it. Drinking too little water can cause some inconvenient problems. That's because clay will draw toxins to it, but like a sponge, if the environment in the digestive channel becomes too dry, it will release these same toxins: "Easy come, easy go." That's when you feel sick and wish you had never eaten the dirt. Drink lots of water, and you will quickly remedy the situation.

If you notice that you get constipated after taking the clay, this is due to a binding of wastes in the colon. Simply take a laxative tea for the first couple of days till you get normal. Thereafter, there should never be a problem with constipation.

A lack of water, interestingly enough, is related to constipation. You need to drink water to get the bowels moving.

Rule 1 is to always drink water. Rule 2 is to drink more of it than you drank obeying Rule 1. Water will help improve your digestion, raise your energy, get your colon moving, and help your clay work. So what are you waiting for? Quench your thirst!

FASTING WITH CLAY

Many books on fasting advise that no vitamins or herbs should be taken during a fast. That's because vitamins will not be properly assimilated, and herbs are food sources. But, whatever the case may be, *clay can safely be taken during a fast*. It will not interfere with the fast. In fact, it will only enhance it.

While I mention throughout the book that clay works as both a food and a medicine, it isn't really one or the other. Clay is clay, not a food or a medicine; it is just a natural substance that performs the functions of both. It should be easy to enjoy the benefits of eating clay because you won't have to worry about violating your fast.

As you probably already know, the main purpose of any fast is to prevent or eliminate disease through body detoxification. Eating the clay on a regular basis throughout a fast will help you to renew your body and see your desired results quicker.

DON'T BE SURPRISED BY THOSE TOXINS

The purpose of any detoxification program is to clean house. Don't be surprised when you begin taking the clay and some "weird" symptoms arise:

- You pass smelly gas.
- Your eliminations are larger than normal.

- Your eliminations are more frequent.
- Your skin breaks out.
- You get weird pains all over your body.
- You start feeling tired.
- You become anxious and nervous.

Every one of these signs points to the fact that your body is cleaning itself out. Most persons will experience symptoms like this to a lesser or greater degree depending on medical history, diet, age, activity level, and overall state of health.

Believe it or not, these symptoms mean that you are well on your way to health. Natural medicine refers to this episode as a "healing crisis" or the symptoms of detoxification. The cells are getting rid of nicotine, caffeine, drugs, pollutants, and many other things. Before these substances are finally eliminated, they run through the bloodstream, causing any number of the symptoms listed above. Typically, any healing crisis will last only one to ten days; then the body evolves to a new stage of health.

In a healing crisis, you may find that, for example, your skin breaks out although you haven't had acne for years. Don't try to stop these symptoms by taking drugs or massive amounts of herbs and vitamins. Simply let them go and allow the body to follow its own course. Your immune system is attempting to revive itself the natural way—by getting rid of the accumulation of poisons (maybe a potential degenerative disease) you've stored in your body for years. Allow the cycle to run without interruption.

Whenever you clean your body expect a detoxification outbreak. It will only last a short while and will hardly inconvenience you. Just as when you clean a floor, expect a little dust to be swept up when you first detoxify. Don't mistakenly think that just because you change your diet for a few meals and begin exercising you will see definite results within days. It took months, or maybe years, for your body to be where it is now. Be fair, and at least give it some time to adjust and work itself out. In the long run, your immune system will be stronger.

The most important thing to know is that when you do experience a healing crisis, you can simply cut back on taking the clay, but do not completely cut it out of your program. Its action will be needed now, more than ever. And when you start feeling healthy, don't be surprised if after a period of time you go through another healing crisis. Health returns in a series of cycles.

PURE OR IMPURE?

If you are concerned about eating clay that has undergone a strict purification process, then look for clays that meet the U.S. federal purity standards for microbial limits, absence of pathogens, absence of adulteration, and product consistency. If the clay you have chosen either does not measure up to this standard or exceeds it, it should not be used. Companies that sell these clays religiously check for the presence of potentially toxic minerals like aluminum and mercury. They make sure there are no overwhelming amounts of certain minerals that could pose potential danger to the system. This purified kind of clay is strongly recommended for everyone, particularly young persons, pregnant women, the elderly, and any persons suffering from a chronic ailment. It is the clay of choice.

It sounds strange that one would even consider eating an unpurified clay, but it's quite common. Many clays sold on the market are not suggested for internal use because they may have unknown numbers of microbes and possible pathogens, but people eat them anyway with good results. A case in point is the green clay imported from southern France. One American company that repackages the clay suggests it should be used only for cosmetic purposes; the reason for this is that this particular green clay has not undergone any sterilzation or purification process. Still, many people purchase this same green clay for internal use and do very well with it.

Further, most health food stores often sell some type of clay in bulk, such as rose clay or jordan clay, for eating. These bulk clays are most often unsterilized, unpurified, and unchecked for mineral consistency.

Because there are so many good clays that have not been tested or purified, it would be difficult for me to recommend that you eat only clays that meet federal purity standards. I make it a habit to switch between both kinds. Many "primitive" people eat clay and do not seem to worry about standards of purity. Animals eat clay and don't bother with that, either.

I suggest that when you are looking for an edible clay, avoid the dirt near your house and purchase the clays sold for internal consumption at a health food store. These are typically the cleanest and most healthful.

Total Body Healing
with Clay

*Everything in Nature contains all the powers of
Nature. Everything is made of one hidden stuff.*

Ralph Waldo Emerson

Health is a natural state of being, active and dynamic, wherein
the individual participates in his or her own well-being. The
body is a complete, self-functioning organism capable of restoring wholeness when it is ill or injured. If there are ob-
stacles that stand in its way to health, it only needs to be
properly and gently stimulated. Once charged, the regenera-
tion processes can begin and health will return. Therefore, the
use of clay can be a part of any wellness program. Clay stimulates the body to do its own healing work and recover from
just about any ailment.

Important: This chapter covers the most common ailments
from acne to gum disease and nausea to ulcers. While clay is
certainly a very effective treatment, it is only one of many
valid therapies. Please do not believe that clay alone can re-
place a good attitude, healthy diet, physical exercise, necessary
supplements, and your doctor's care and advice.

THE DIGESTIVE SYSTEM

It would take too much time to refer to every digestive ailment clay treats; if I did, the information would be repetitive and tedious. Clay is noted to be of great benefit to *any gastrointestinal disorder*. Naturopaths and herbalists have prescribed clay for its chemical and mechanical actions for many ailments including gastritis, Crohn's disease, and irritable bowel syndrome, and even to help protect against bowel cancer. But remember, clay is not a drug, nor does it work like one. Clay binds with and removes body toxins in the stomach, small intestine, and colon. It also stimulates the normal mechanism of the intestinal tract. In this way, it activates the immune system to defend itself against illness caused by too long an exposure to harmful poisons that accumulate in the bowel.

Bad Breath

Clay has often been referred to as an internal mouthwash. That's because taking the clay daily will help to relieve the digestive tract, supporting elimination and binding the poisons that may be the cause of the unpleasant smell. This collection of poisons is likely the root of bad breath. Therefore, the channels of elimination must be activated. Once they are clean, there will be no bad odor to escape through the mouth. Try taking one teaspoon of clay per day added to a full glass of water.

Constipation

When the bowels do not move properly, the reasons are usually improper diet, lack of fiber, lack of water, and faulty digestion. The first thing to do is drink lots of water—no other liquids, just water. That will help the clay to work and get the system normalized.

Clay produces desirable bulk in the intestinal tract, which in turn stimulates normal intestinal motions and contractions that move food substances in the intestine. Therefore, it can help protect against chronic constipation. Clay is not a laxative, however. Laxatives work by irritating the mucous membranes, causing the colon to contract. This in time exhausts the muscles, but clay does not irritate the muscles.

Begin taking the clay once a day on an empty stomach before retiring to bed. Allow the clay at least one to seven days to regulate the system; thereafter, eat it on a maintenance dose.

A word to the wise: If you drink an adequate amount of water when taking the clay, the constipation will likely be eased. In the beginning, you may want to support your clay with the herbs cascara sagrada and Chinese rhubarb root, which help tone the bowels and support bowel function. Any health food store will carry either of these herbs in a variety of forms: packaged singly or in combination with other herbs. Follow the directions on the bottle.

Diarrhea

Clay is recognized worldwide as a treatment for diarrhea. In China, clay was used for many centuries as a cure for summer diarrhea and cholera. In 1712, Father Deutrecolle, a Jesuit missionary traveling through China, described the clay works there and mentioned that clay was used in treating diarrhea. In fact, as late as 1919, clay proved an invaluable medicine in the cholera epidemic that swept through China.

In times of war, clay has been an outstanding medicine for its healing capabilities. During World War II, French soldiers ate clay to combat dysentery. The use of clay with other medications during the Balkan war of 1910 reduced the mortality from cholera among the soldiers from a high 60 percent to an unbelievably low 3 percent!

Clay has also been used as an adsorptive in the symptomatic treatment of various forms of enteritis, including ulcerative colitis.

Gastrointestinal adsorbents, including clay, are presently recommended for acute diarrhea and bacillary dysentery to adsorb the toxins that produce the diarrhea. Clay has been used in the treatment of abnormal intestinal fermentation to adsorb gases, toxins, and bacteria. In a fluid medium, it carries down large numbers of bacteria and adsorbs the toxins of cholera, typhoid, dysentery, and, apparently, the putrefactive and proteolytic bacteria.

Investigations have indicated that smectite clay adsorbs certain viruses, including those of intestinal influenza. The fastest results were observed in intestinal influenza, in which the diarrhea was controlled in an average of 2.2 days. Smectite clay has antiviral properties.

The clay should be taken frequently: two tablespoons added to water, three times per day. The condition responds better to quick, continued treatment, so repeat the dose often (every two to four hours). When the symptoms disappear, stay on a maintenance dose of one tablespoon a day.

For infants who suffer from diarrhea, add one-half teaspoon of clay to the bottle and shake vigorously. It will mix with the solution, and the infant won't even know it's there.

A study of the therapeutic efficacy of clay for acute diarrhea of diverse causes was reported in the *Medical Annals of the District of Columbia* (Damrau 1961). The causes were virus infection, food allergy, spastic colitis, mucous colitis, and food poisoning. The symptoms evaluated in 35 cases in addition to diarrhea, included abdominal cramps, anorexia, malaise, headache, nausea, and weakness.

The group included 25 women and 10 men. Every effort was made to obtain a homogeneous group of patients so as to eliminate variables from the study.

As a standard treatment, two tablespoons of smectite clay in distilled water were given three times daily. In cases of food allergy, the dosage was increased to more than six tablespoonfuls daily.

Acute diarrhea was relieved by clay in 34 of the 35 cases (97 percent) in an average time of 3.8 days, and the number of daily bowel movements was reduced to an average of 1.8.

In the 18 cases of diarrhea due to virus infection, the therapeutic response was unusually prompt. In the 8 cases due to food allergy, the diarrhea persisted longer and on many occasions returned if the same allergenic food was eaten again.

The concomitant symptoms of abdominal cramps, anorexia, malaise, headache, nausea, and weakness were also relieved. No side effects attributable to the medication were observed in any case.

Diverticulosis

When the colon is not properly emptied, the walls of the intestines form balloons, or diverticula. Soon, undigested food creeps into the pouches and may cause inflammation. The condition, known as diverticulosis, is mainly due to constipation. The clay may be taken frequently to prevent this.

However, if you have already been stricken by the ailment, and you have never taken clay, it is safe to do so. Your doctor may recommend a three-day juice fast to accelerate the healing process. While you fast, take two tablespoons of clay twice per day to adsorb toxins and accelerate the elimination of intestinal waste. Eating clay will also help to form soft stool, which relieves the need to strain.

After you have finished the fast, keep taking the clay and follow up with the proper health regimen.

Note: Before starting a fast, consult your physician.

Irritable Bowel Syndrome

This ailment is characterized by alternating conditions of diarrhea and constipation with gas, pain, and emotional ups and downs. Because the cause of irritable bowel syndrome is unknown, treating the condition with drugs can be dangerous. Even naturopathic doctors have a difficult time in controlling, managing, and curing the disease.

I suggest one heaping teaspoon of clay three times per day and at bedtime. After visible results, drop the frequency down to once per day. The clay should be taken on an empty stomach so it will not interfere with the digestion of food.

Nausea and Vomiting (and Food Poisoning)

Clay has proved itself beneficial in the relief of nausea and vomiting. It is an excellent treatment for morning sickness (see chapter 8, Clay and Pregnancy) and food poisoning. In India, clay was found useful in the treatment of acute bacterial food poisonings in the British Army.

In cases of nausea, vomiting, and suspected food poisoning, take one teaspoon of clay every two hours as long as needed. Drink plenty of water to help the clay absorb/adsorb the toxins, bacteria, or viruses that are causing the nausea. If the nausea is especially severe, one teaspoon every ten minutes will be helpful. Usually, four teaspoons is enough to halt the symptoms; typically, the nausea will cease within one hour. Thereafter, you can follow up with one dose every four hours until bedtime. This will help to further relieve the gastrointestinal tract and take a heavy burden off the liver. Helpful herb teas include peppermint, ginger, and alfalfa. Ipecacuanha and nux vomica are supporting homeopathic remedies.

In addition, the clay is a preferred treatment for any gastrointestinal infections caused by *E. coli, Shigella, Salmonella,* and *Klebsiella,* in the same dosages as given above.

Overweight and Undernourished: Clay As a Slimming Agent

You may have come into contact with a hundred diet products and programs, but I'll bet you've never before heard of clay being used as a slimming agent. All over the world, people ingest clay to help acquire and maintain a shapely figure. Sound strange? Earlier I mentioned that clay is typically ingested in famine times to help combat starvation; it temporarily satisfies the hunger and creates a feeling of fullness. For this same reason, clay will keep the weight off. It expands in the stomach, making less room for the food, and thereby relieves the pangs of hunger.

The advantage to taking clay for weight loss is that it helps to increase the number of bowel movements as well as their quality. Often the weight of waste matter alone is enough to add a few extra pounds to the body. For instance, many of the various diet products on the market contain laxatives to help relieve a constipated condition. Furthermore, clay will assist the assimilation of food. This may, in turn, cut down on the intense need to eat, which may be a cause of malnourishment. Even in an overweight person, if the cells are not having their nutritional needs met, the body can starve to death.

When dieting with clay, the important thing to watch out for is that you don't skip meals or skip out on good nutrition. While the clay helps to satisfy hunger, it doesn't work the same as a "fat burner." It's not going to blast you with a caffeine high and enable you to drop pounds quickly. Therefore, it would be good for you to include some other diet supplements in your program, such as a citrin or chromium picolinate, for greater benefit.

The recommended dosage of clay is one heaping teaspoon taken an hour before meals in an eight-ounce glass of water or juice. Try mixing it with a green drink like Greens Plus or Kyo-Green for improved results.

Parasites

Parasites are taken more seriously now than ever before in the United States. The risk of parasitic infection is growing. You may have heard of the *Cryptosporidium,* an intestinal parasite that spreads by contact with infected feces: anything from diapers to water tainted by farm runoff. In Milwaukee, it found its way into the water and sickened an estimated 400,000 people. It is frequently found overseas and is becoming an increasing problem for AIDS patients and day-care centers here.

While many herbs and homeopathic remedies are suggested for this condition, I believe clay offers one of the finest treatments for all types of parasites. First, its use will stimulate the gall bladder to increase the flow of bile according to Raymond Dextreit, a French naturopath. He writes that no parasite can live too long under any bilious condition.

Second, considerable research has shed light on the connection between clay eating and parasites. The *American Journal of Clinical Nutrition* mentioned this in a recent article: "Geophagy can be a source of nutrients. Its primary way of enhancing nutritional status appears to be, however, to counter dietary toxins and, secondarily, *the effects of gastrointestinal parasites* [italics mine]" (Johns and Duquette 1991). Further, numerous citations in a host of other journals collaborate this fact: throughout the globe, people eat clay in response to parasites, but not only gastrointestinal parasites.

Third, worms are themselves clay-eaters and are attracted to clay. As a result, when the clay is eliminated from the body, so are the worms. But the process isn't quick; for every worm eliminated several eggs are usually left behind. However, the eggs hatch, the new worms are also immediately attracted to the clay, and in time, the entire problem should be disposed of.

Poisoning

The *American Journal of Medicine* published a study conducted with Paraquat, a widely used herbicide, in an effort to understand how medicinal therapy can help avoid a fatal outcome. Doctors fed lethal doses of the herbicide to rats and recorded the effects. They noted that an excess of the poison caused respiratory failure, liver damage, and kidney failure, which soon led to death.

Several adsorbents were shown to be effective in counteracting the effects of the poison before the poison was ingested. Among them were bentonite and Fuller's earth, commonly called montmorillonite. However, only one adsorbent proved successful in counteracting the toxic effects of the poison *after* it was ingested: montmorillonite clay.

In this experimental situation, clay was given in repeated doses rather than single doses. The effectiveness of repeated doses is apparently due to its ability to prevent the gastrointestinal absorption of Paraquat, which can continue up to 30 hours after ingestion in rats. Surprisingly, even when the treatment was delayed for 10 hours after the oral administration of Paraquat, the therapy was successful. The rats did not die and toxic damage was minimal.

The authors of the report went on to say that since urinary Paraquat levels have been detected for as long as 31 days after ingestion, continued efforts, as well as early efforts, to eliminate absorbed Paraquat may be important. Therefore, continual use of the clay is advisable because of its ongoing adsorptive properties. The doctors concluded the article by saying that in case any lethal doses of Paraquat are ingested, Fuller's earth should be administered as soon as possible.

In cases of gastrointestinal poisoning, one teaspoon of clay can be repeated at regular intervals (every 1 to 2 hours) up to 48 hours after ingestion. If the case is severe and serious, please go to the emergency room!

Note: Robert Robertson, author of *Fuller's Earth*, has a very interesting comment on the role of clay as an antidote to poison. He writes,

> Although the use of Fuller's earth (calcium montmorillonite) as an antidote to poisons has been known for centuries, and the scientific reasons for its success have been known for decades, it is strange that, in a world where heavy metal solutions, alkaloids, cationic pesticides and detergents could be accidentally ingested, Fuller's earth is not yet included in Red Cross or First Aid Boxes, in factories, homes and chemical laboratories.

Ulcers

In Russia, smectite clay has been used in the therapy of peptic ulcer. That's because clay helps to alkalinize an acid stomach. It will also rebuild the gastrointestinal wall that has been eaten through by the acid. Again, the clay must be a smectite (montmorillonite), because not all clay will heal an ulcer. The

mineral must contain a sufficient amount of the elements sodium and calcium, otherwise it will not be effective. It works
by absorbing the ions in excess (hydrogen, in this case) and,
in exchange, giving off the sodium and calcium to effectively
neutralize the acid.

One teaspoon can be taken twice per day and as needed—
that is, if the ulcer suddenly flares up. The clay can be mixed
with aloe vera gel for quick relief and long-term curative
results.

LIVER PROBLEMS

The liver is frequently referred to as the body's detoxification
pilot. It breaks down poisons or transforms them into less
harmful compounds. The poisons include toxins found in food
(nitrates, monosodium glutamate, and herbicides), toxins produced by the body (ketones, indoles, phenols, and aldehydes),
as well as toxins in the environment. In addition, the liver
performs a long list of other functions, including the manufacture of bile salts, the activation of vitamin D, and storage of
glycogen, vitamin A, copper, and iron. The liver, without a
doubt, is absolutely vital to one's health.

Clay can be an invaluable aid to a poorly functioning
liver. It works indirectly on the organ, as follows. After you
eat, the absorption of nutrients takes place throughout the
length of the small intestine and the large intestine. From here
they are transported in the bloodstream to the liver by way of
the hepatic portal system (the flow of blood from the digestive
organs to the liver). After their passage through the liver, they
move through the heart and then enter general circulation.

If the bowels are not working right, waste matter will be
continually reabsorbed into the blood stream and carried to
the liver. As a result, the liver is forced into doing extra work

that might not be needed if the bowels were in good working condition. This places an unnecessary burden on the liver and the rest of the body. Eating clay will have an indirect positive effect on the liver by facilitating the cleansing of the gastrointestinal tract. Through adsorption and absorption, many of the toxins will exit directly through the colon and bypass the liver and general circulation. Further, because immune function is governed by the Kupffer cells of the liver, which in turn respond to the chemical balance of the colon, intestinal health is integral to quality liver function. Although clay does not work directly on the organ, its actions are soon felt there.

Allergies and Hay Fever

Allergies and hay fever are caused by the release of histamines. The liver becomes plugged up with toxins and fatty tissue and therefore cannot produce the necessary antihistamines to neutralize the allergic reactions. The first thing to do is clean and rebuild the liver. Once that is done, the allergies and hay fever may disappear.

The good news about clay is that not only will it help stimulate the eliminatory channels, but it can effectively treat allergies and hay fever. Adsorption is a relatively quick process—almost instantaneous in certain cases. The adsorptive surfaces of the clay prevent the allergic reaction by quickly neutralizing allergens before these foreign invaders can attach themselves to the blood cells. In addition, any histamines produced by the allergens that have "gotten away" can also be quickly adsorbed. Water-soluble allergens are bound up by the clay because of its intense hydrophilic (water-loving) nature.

Some people, after taking the clay, notice an immediate improvement in their condition. Sometimes the allergies and hay fever disappear altogether. Others see no sudden improvement and must keep taking the clay quite a while before they obtain visible results. The reaction, of course, depends on the state of the liver and the condition of the immune system. A healthier liver will bounce back more quickly than one that is sick.

If you do not achieve results relatively quickly, then give the clay time to work. One heaping teaspoon once per day in a glass of freshly squeezed lemon water will be sufficient. In the meantime, take advantage of homeopathic detoxification remedies and herbal formulas to stimulate cleansing.

Note: Hives are a skin rash that is typically due to an allergic reaction. The same suggestions for allergies and hay fever can be applied in this case. In addition, see The Skin: A Channel of Elimination, below.

Anemia

Clay is frequently used to influence anemia because of the relation of anemia to the liver; anthropologists confirm this practice among various cultures across the globe. The liver purifies the blood and gives it most of the nutritive elements it needs and increases the number of red blood cells and regularizes their iron content.

Most clays provide both ferrous and ferric iron in an easily assimilated form. It should be noted, however, that "although iron deficiency has been established in some forms of pica, no clear evidence has been presented to link geophagy and iron need" (Johns and Duquette 1991). The debate over whether or not clay is suitable for treating anemia is unresolved.

Try one heaping teaspoon of clay three times per day, on an empty stomach. In addition, eat as many iron-rich foods, such as spinach or parsley, and chlorophyll as you can. These are important to the formation of red blood cells. While clay may help with anemia, a change in diet also is very important. Consult your physician for treatment.

Hepatitis and Cirrhosis

Clay can be very valuable in the treatment of hepatitis and cirrhosis. Most persons in the natural health field recommend an immediate cleansing through fasting and purging. For one week, if possible, nothing should be taken except distilled water and fruit and vegetable juices. Check with your doctor, however, before you embark on any new program, especially a fast. If you want more information on fasting, any book on cleansing will outline a complete program. Many authors stress that supplement intake is not advised during the cleansing process, but often they fail to mention ingesting clay. Although dirt eating has been around since time immemorial, most people today are not aware of geophagy as a medicinal treatment and therefore fail to take it into consideration. As I repeated earlier in the book, it is okay to take clay daily during a fast.

Eat three tablespoons of clay per day, in addition to following a doctor-recommended program, until your condition stabilizes. Simply dissolve one tablespoon in water (juice is fine, particularly freshly squeezed lemon juice with no added sugar). Thereafter, follow up with one heaping teaspoon twice per day. In addition, clay packs applied daily to the liver area are helpful. Edgar Cayce advises applying cod liver oil packs. Both can be alternated. Refer to The Physical Application of Clay, below.

THE SKIN: A CHANNEL OF ELIMINATION

The condition of the skin is a good indication of what is happening inside the body. Most people are not aware that the skin is the largest organ and a means of eliminating waste; each day waste passes through the pores of the skin.

Everything that affects the body in turn affects the skin. When the body is full of toxic wastes and cannot eliminate them properly, various skin ailments may result. The only effective way to get rid of these conditions is by cleaning the body inside and out.

Acne

Most acne is relatively easy to treat with the right methods—usually, a good diet and the daily ingestion of clay. My younger teenage brother got rid of bad acne within one week of eating clay. At first he said it wasn't doing too much for his skin. Then, out of the blue, he called me and frantically asked me to bring over another jar of "dirt." He had run out of the clay for a couple of days, and his pimples returned.

The clay enriches and cleanses the blood, promoting better circulation and allowing the skin to get rid of waste. Take one teaspoon of clay twice per day. Mix with lemon water for best results. Also, prepare daily a detoxification tea containing red clover, burdock, sarsaparilla, parsley, and milk thistle. These herbs will help encourage healing.

If clay ingestion helps only partially, use the clay as a masque also. The best clay for this purpose is kaolinite or jordan clay. I mix essential oils with clay to make a mud that will clean up, tone, and invigorate the most affected skin. These oils include lemon, tea tree, carrot seed, and bergamot. I encourage you to work with the oils and try blending your own. In any case, the masque is a great addition to clay consumption. See The Physical Application of Clay, below.

Eczema, Itching, Hives

These are the most common skin complaints. The same health program must be followed for each irritation if the body is to get rid of the problem at hand. First, consider a detoxification program consisting of natural supplements such as milk thistle, N-acetyl-cysteine, glutathione, and alfalfa juice concentrate. Second, take hot baths to help open the pores of the skin. Last, take one tablespoon of clay once or twice per day, preferably on rising, one hour before your breakfast, and on an empty stomach before you go to bed. Apply clay packs to the affected area as well.

THE PHYSICAL APPLICATION OF CLAY

This book focuses mainly on the benefits of eating clay. I do not cover the physical application of clay to a large extent because most of that information has been laid out in two excellent books: *Our Earth, Our Cure* by Raymond Dextreit, and *The Healing Clay,* by Michael Abehsera. These books describe the proper application of clay packs to treat such conditions as headaches, lumbago, hernia, ulcers, burns, boils, varicose veins, and ear infections.

The Clay Pack

The clay pack may be used to treat neuritis, sciatica (a large pack over the hips and abdomen is advised for this), local pains and inflammations, and patches of skin disease. The following method can be used to prepare a clay pack:

1. Mix clay with water to make a thick paste.
2. Spread evenly on the back of a cloth or gauze (preferably a thick layer of clay).

3. Apply to affected area and hold in place. Renew as
   often as necessary.

Clay possesses an antibacterial action as well as an anti-
septic action. Therefore, for just about any skin ailment, clay
will stop the growth of bacteria, prevent decay, and arrest the
development of microorganisms. This is why, for example, it
is so effective in the treatment of acne, boils, and wounds.
Also, clay packs may be useful as an auxiliary remedy while
healing broken bones, strains, and sprains, because they are
said to help reconstruct damaged tissue.

Clay Ointment

Take a lump of clay and soak it in cold water for two hours.
Pour off the water and remove any gravel or foreign substances. Next, add tea made from any of the following herbs:
St. John's wort, yellow dock, or horsetail. To prepare the tea,
simmer an ounce of the chosen herb in a pint of water for 10
to 15 minutes, and strain. Then, add enough tea to clay to
create an ointment. This preparation can be applied liberally
to any ulcer or sore. It should be renewed every four to six
hours depending on the severity and the amount of discharge.
You may wish to apply the ointment before bedtime and let
it remain throughout the night.

Clay Masque

The clay facial masque deep-cleans pores, exfoliates dead cells,
and leaves the skin feeling soft and clean. It stimulates skin
circulation and has an astringent action on sagging tissues.
The facial muscles become toned from the application of the
clay masque.

You may wish to use clay alone when preparing a masque, or mix it with several other ingredients. One formula consists of three ounces of clay, one egg, and equal parts of honey and cold water. The amount of honey added determines the hydrating ability of the masque. Persons with dry skin, or those who live in a dry climate, should add more honey than water. Persons with oily skin, or those who live in a humid climate, may prefer less honey and more water for a more absorbent masque. Leave the masque on for about 20 minutes, then rinse, rub, or brush off. After preparing the masque, you can store what is left over in the refrigerator.

The Clay Bath

The clay bath has been much talked about lately; you may already have heard of it. It is a fairly simple procedure, and it can do a lot of good in a realtively short time. Because of clay's excellent drawing effect, the clay has the power to literally pull out toxicities through the pores of the skin in the bath.

It is a very simple procedure to prepare the clay bath. Adding four pounds of bentonite clay (you probably will not want to use an expensive, edible montmorillonite) to your bathtub. Pour the clay very slowly, at the point of the faucet, into the running warm water. Using a spoon or a wire wisk, stir the water to keep the clay particles from sticking together.

Stay in the tub for 20 to 25 minutes. Then stand up, and rinse yourself underneath the shower. Do not drain the tub just yet. This clay solution must sit for a little time (not more than three or four hours) in order to settle to the bottom. At this point you have several choices. You can now drain the tub, which is not recommended because that would clog the drain. It's better to skim off the surface water and pour it down the sink; when you're finished, compost it or toss it into your yard.

After skimming the water, you may want to take a peek at the clay. Some people say that the clay at the bottom of the bathtub changes color, sometimes becoming a dark brown or black. This is a supposed result of the absorbed and adsorbed toxins. Others say that you should not handle the leftover clay with your hands; instead, you must use rubber gloves when scooping it out because you are at risk of chemical burn because the clay is now supposed to be very toxic.

My experience with the clay leads me to believe that depending on the type of mineral clay used for the bath, it may very possibly change hues. However, the clays I have used for the bath have never shown this quality. As for being unable to touch the clay because of a potentially high burn risk . . . well, I doubt that. It seems implausible to me that one's body would release toxicities capable of burning one's hands within 20 minutes.

Other Applications of Clay

Additional uses for clay include the following:

1. *As a shower scrub in place of soap.* Mix with water in the palm of your hand. Rinse off.
2. *As a body masque.* Apply to the neck, shoulders, breasts, arms, legs, and feet. Apply as a paste and allow it to dry. Rinse off.
3. *As an exfoliating body masque.* Instead of rinsing it off, rub or brush off the masque when it is dry to remove even more dead skin and to stimulate circulation.
4. *For sunburn, burns, and scalds.* Apply a paste to help take out the redness and relieve the pain.

5. *For insect bites and stings.* Apply as a paste and allow it to dry. Then, rinse it off and renew the pack.

6. *For sore feet and/or body.* The clay can be added to a foot soak or the bath water for added relaxation.

CIRCULATORY PROBLEMS

The Heart and Blood

According to Michael Abehsara, author of *The Healing Clay,* clay is rich in diastases (enzymes), which account for its ability to fix free oxygen and purify and enrich the blood. Free radicals are atoms whose electrons have been stripped; while a certain number of them are necessary to stave off invading bacteria, too many can attack the body, causing cellular breakdown. Clay contributes to an improved blood supply.

High levels of blood risk factors, such as too many free radicals, help to explain the breakdown of the cardiovascular system in the form of strokes or heart attacks. If the body continues to pump dirty blood to the heart, heart disease is sure to follow. The vessel walls are eventually weakened by weak blood, which cannot carry the nutrients needed for blood vessel reinforcement. Clay's cleansing action on the stomach, small intestine, and colon may prevent this.

The suggested dosage is one level tablespoon once per day, taken together with fiber (psyllium seed, apple pectin, or guar gum). Fiber, too, is known to reduce the level of cholesterol in the blood. Like the clay, it binds to the bile. The Arabs of old, in Persia, took clay to "fortify" the heart.

Hemorrhoids

Hemorrhoids are varicose veins in the anal area, possibly resulting from pushing and straining when going to the bathroom; they are also related to hepatic congestion. You can try taking clay internally for this condition, one tablespoon once per day. Next, follow up with the application of clay packs. While the clay is effective in treatment, the process is slow, and it can therefore afford the help of other healing agents such as the herb collinsia root, or any of the following homeopathic remedies: aloe socotrina, nux vomica, hamemelis virginica, or calendula gel.

FOR WOMEN ONLY: MENSTRUAL CRAMPS

Eating clay is therapeutic in cases of menstrual cramps. By drawing the metabolic waste products and improving intestinal health, clay helps prevent cramps and lessen the related symptoms (headaches, bloating, irritability). Many naturopaths agree that menstrual cramps are not only a hormonal matter, but are partly due to constipation. One teaspoon of clay taken twice per day in prune juice will be helpful.

FOR MEN ONLY: PROSTATE PROBLEMS

The prostate is located between the rectum and the neck of the bladder. Because of its location, its health can be directly influenced by the condition of the bowels. An impacted colon will undoubtedly affect the health of the prostate. Therefore, a cleansing program is the first thing to implement in any prostate rebuilding program.

Clay will help to prevent the accumulation of waste matter and feces that can clog up the rectum. This could help to diminish the possibility of any future prostate problems, or remedy a current one. One tablespoon taken once per day on an empty stomach will be all that is needed. In a case of BPH (benign prostatic hypertrophy), the clay should be taken daily in addition to standard herbs like pygeum, saw palmetto, and ginseng.

COMMON AILMENTS

Arthritis and Rheumatic Symptoms

Some arthritic problems are mainly due to an accumulation of waste matter that has settled in specific areas of the body such as the knee, hand, and lower back. Sometimes, uric acid is the culprit and will attack the cartilage of the joints, the tendons, or other tissues.

In cases of arthritis, the clay's action is entirely indirect. Because of a lack of scientific evidence documenting the effectiveness of clay against arthritis, I only write this section as a testimony to some individuals who have been assisted by the clay. When taken internally, clay may help to relieve the pain, reduce stiffness, and increase joint motion.

One heaping teaspoon of clay should be taken twice per day, added to water or juice. Incorporate other supplements into your program such as glucosamine/chondroitin sulfate, shark cartilage, or cetyl myristoleate, because clay tends to function better when thoughtfully combined with other remedies. In addition, you may apply packs to the affected area to speed desired results. Refer to The Physical Application of Clay, above. Remember that the clay must be taken separately from these cartilegenous precursors to be properly absorbed.

Chronic Fatigue Syndrome

Recent research from Temple University suggests that a blood marker from chronic fatigue syndrome (CFS) may soon be available. Researchers have isolated a specific antiviral pathway that consistently demonstrates disruption in immune function.

A low-density enzyme unique to people with CSF is the suspected culprit. In chronic fatigue syndrome, RNA (ribonucleic acid) function in the body becomes disrupted, inhibiting protein synthesis. This causes various symptoms, such as tiredness, aches and pains, delayed muscle recovery, and mood swings. CFS is referred to as a complex illness, because of the many symptoms it produces.

Proper rest is essential to the successful treatment of CFS, but the right balance of activity is also crucial. Absolute inactivity can result in a deconditioned state. On the other hand, becoming too active may overextend the muscles, thus delaying chances for recovery. Therefore, people with this condition must avoid strenuous activity and must treat the sleep disorder, so common in this condition, that may further aggravate the muscle pain. For people with CFS, sometimes the prescribed medications for sleep are more effective than melatonin or herbs like valerian and kava kava.

Until effective medications are made available, people with this disorder must take a host-centered approach to the illness: stimulating the body's own forces of healing through lifestyle changes may, over time, bring about recovery. Detoxification is obviously needed. Since immune function is governed by the Kupffer cells of the liver, which in turn respond to the chemical balance of the colon, rebalancing the chemical state of the colon is necessary. In other words, keeping the gut clear will assist in combating the deleterious effects of the disease. Clay should be taken daily to absorb bodily toxins and ensure intestinal health.

Often several viruses and fungi are activated in cases of CFS. For instance, many people who come down with the illness are diagnosed with Candida in the gut. According to an article in the *Canadian Journal of Microbiology,* clay has the capacity to adsorb and eliminate viruses (Lipson and Stolzky 1985).

Anyone with CFS is advised to be open to all methods of treatment. Taking clay has its advantages, one being its ability to act as a pattern and catalyst for the formation of long peptide chains. It is hoped that, in the future, more light will be shed on this subject. In addition to clay, the following nutritional supplements will be of use to anyone battling CFS: coenzyme Q_{10}, magnesium, malic acid, quercitin, bromelain, lentinus edodes (shiitake) mycelia extract (LEM), antioxidants, vitamin B_{12}, and the other B-complex vitamins. The dose of each supplement varies according to the individual constitution; therefore, it would be wise to seek the advice of a health professional.

Take one heaping teaspoon of clay twice a day in juice or water. Expect the clay treatment to take time; the results are not instantaneous.

Most people diagnosed with CFS who begin taking clay see results of some kind in 7 to 30 days.

Gum Disease: Gingivitis and Pyorrhea

The clay treatments for gingivitis and pyorrhea are the same (gingivitis will develop into pyorrhea if not taken care of). The first line of action involves brushing the teeth three times a week with clay. If you cannot find a toothpaste containing clay (available at most health food stores), then use clay powder. Mix the powder with sea salt or baking soda until it reaches a paste consistency. The clay is absorbent, so it will not be abrasive, and it helps harden the enamel while it aids in gum tissue repair. Furthermore, if used regularly, it helps to prevent gum recession. On the other days, switch to a natural toothpaste. If you feel the need to get fluoride, many natural toothpastes contain this ingredient.

Next, prepare clay balls or "clay chew" (see page 98) to

be taken throughout the day. The clay possesses antibacterial properties. A good time to apply the clay chew is at night before you go to bed. In this way, you can be assured that the clay will stay in continued contact with the gums. When you wake up in the morning, you will have swallowed the clay and it will be gone. Don't forget to massage your gums.

In Oaxaca, Mexico, clay is a substitute for tooth powder, and its users maintain that it helps keep their teeth white.

Headaches

Because headaches are rooted in many causes, the approach to the symptoms must be host-centered. If the problem is due in part to chemical sensitivities, food allergies, or the circulation of toxins, the clay will enable the body to detoxify more efficiently and utilize nutrients more effectively.

Syphilis

It seems strange to include a venereal disease in a book of this nature. Yet, believe it or not, among specific cultures, clay eating is a cure for syphilis. I don't know why that is, or in what respect it works. I don't know anyone who either has or has had syphilis who ever ate clay, so I don't know how long the cure takes, or whether clay really does cure. Most so-called primitive cultures offer no explanation for how a mineral clay works on syphilis—they are content just to say it does. And the anthropologists are content to record the information.

ADDITIONAL USES

- Add clay powder to water for its purification properties (whenever I visit Mexico, I bring a jar of clay with me and add a pinch or two to every glass of water I drink).

- Add clay powder to your dog's or cat's water bowl.
- Clay can be added to aquariums to control the growth of algae.
- Clay minerals provide an excellent source of nutrients for plants, and also adsorb many free mineral ions in the soil. Add to the soil freely.
- Clay helps to control insects (diatomaceous earth). Add to the soil.
- Use clay to remove mildew from bathroom tiles.

Clay and Pregnancy

> *A pilgrim from El Salvador and her grown-up*
> *daughter browsing among the market stalls around*
> *the basilica enthusiastically claimed that they ate*
> *the holy tablets [clay], and when asked, "Do they*
> *do you any good?" the woman's sparkling eyes and*
> *instant response was: "Of course they do: I have*
> *eight children!"*
>
> John M. Hunter and Oscar H. Horst,
> *National Geographic Research*

A mother-to-be sometimes has strange cravings. For no apparent reason, her body suddenly feels starved for certain inedible substances such as charcoal, chalk, or plain dirt. She will go out of her way to eat them, sneaking into the backyard to scoop up a tiny bit of mud in her hand to suck on, or running into the front yard to peel bark off a tree and chew it as if it were a piece of gum. If you ask her why she does this, she may shrug or say, "I don't know, no special reason," or she might say, "I just like it."

Even though these pregnant earth-eaters may not be able to explain their reasons, I believe their actions hold a purpose. Intuitively, the body makes its needs known through physical cravings. When they are responded to, our bodies are "fulfilled" and we are compensated with health. In this case, the mother and her newborn are rewarded.

Well, here's good news for those mothers who run to the

backyard to grab a handful of clay but don't know why: there is a type of dirt they can safely eat—clay. Clay eating is most common during pregnancy, and it is said to be the most favorable practice a mother can undertake for herself and her unborn child.

A Present for You and the Baby

The following reports explain the many uses of clay by pregnant women everywhere.

Before Pregnancy

- Eaten by women who want to bear children. The clay is supposed to have an effect during normal menstruation, before conception has occurred. It is taken as a means of encouraging future pregnancy.
- Recommended for women who are sterile.
- Good for cleaning the body, creating a better environment to house an infant.

During Pregnancy

- It is believed that the unborn infant likes it.
- Promotes healthy digestion.
- Prevents and/or counteracts morning sickness.
- Among the women in one culture, it is thought the fetus will be bigger if the mother eats clay.
- Helps with minor discomforts.
- People in some cultures believe the clay ensures that the child will have a dark complexion; others, a light complexion.
- Has mineral nutrient contents. Many women insist

that clay provides calcium.
- Gives the fetus "good bones and teeth."
- Protects against any unfortunate mishap during pregnancy.
- Montmorillonite clay will calm stomach acidity.
- Montmorillonite clay adsorbs metabolic toxins such as steroidal metabolites associated with pregnancy.

Delivery

- The clay is placed on the tongue of a woman in the belief it facilitates delivery and expulsion of the afterbirth.
- The fetus rises in the womb, making delivery easier.
- Clay eases labor pains, accelerates the delivery, and strengthens the expectant mother.

Breastfeeding

- Women rub their breasts with a paste made from clay to stimulate the secretion of milk.
- Taken internally, it is considered good for lactation.

Hold Your Horses! Is This Safe?

Before I go on any further, you may already be wondering, "That's fine that so many women take clay. But how do I know it is really safe for me and my child?"

Yes, clay eating is a safe and suitable practice that can be maintained during pregnancy. But, as I have emphasized throughout the book, it is important to find the *right* clay. Not all clays are good for eating. Take a clay that meets the stringent U.S. federal purity standards (see chapter 6). You will want a clay whose label says "montmorillonite." This clay would be the best clay for your needs. Some purified bentonites on the market are also of excellent quality.

How Do I Take the Clay?

In taking clay when you are pregnant, there is no major difference from taking it at other times. For safety reasons, here are a few guidelines:

1. You must pay particular attention to the clay you are about to eat. What kind of mineral clay is it?
2. Have someone sample it for you. Watch its effects on that person—that will help you know what the clay will do for you. Pick someone who is not pregnant, obviously, and have that person eat the clay for at least two weeks daily.
3. When you are sure the clay is okay for digestion, begin slowly:

- Start with $1/8$ teaspoon per day the first week.
- $1/4$ teaspoon per day the second week.
- $1/2$ teaspoon per day the third week.
- 1 teaspoon per day the fourth week.
- Thereafter, adjust the dosage as needed, adding more or less. Listen to your body.

When Shall I Take the Clay?

Women in different cultures eat clay at different stages of pregnancy. The women of Nigeria eat earth during the first three months of pregnancy. Women in other cultures eat clay only in the most advanced stages of pregnancy. Still others practice eating clay throughout the entire pregnancy and even during breastfeeding. Eating habits vary according to the culture and the type of clay. Consult your health professional for a recommended time frame.

Note: Because of the seriousness of pregnancy, please consult your health professional before embarking on any new program.

I'm Ready to Eat Dirt

Health that mocks the doctor's rules,
Knowledge never learned of schools.

John Greenleaf Whittier

WHICH CLAY DO I BUY?

In chapter 3, we discussed the disparity among mineral clays—
that clays may be incorrectly labeled under a name, yet the
label may not be indicative of its true mineral contents. For
instance, a beautiful bottle with pretty designs might say
"montmorillonite" but contain only 50 percent of this mineral. The rest could likely be made up of other minerals, such
as illite and chlorite.

If you are looking to purchase an authentic, pure montmorillonite, how do you know which clay to choose? This is
an important question, since not all companies submit their
clays to high standards of purification and consistency.

Picking a clay is really a matter of prudence more than
anything else. Talk to the employees in the health food store
and ask them which edible clays sell best. Don't be afraid to
ask them questions. They work with these products all the

93

time, and they will be happy to help you pick the product to fit your needs. Here are some questions to consider asking when looking for clay:

- Which clay sells the best?
- Which clay do customers return to purchase more of? (Chances are that if no one comes back for the product, it generally is not worth buying.)
- Has the management had any complaints about any of these particular clays?
- Have you ever taken any of these clay products? If you have, could you tell me about them?
- Which companies selling clay are among the strongest and most reputable in the industry?
- Do you have any literature on any of these clay products? (Stores get tons of literature all the time; unless they throw it away, you may be able to find some useful information written by the supplier.)
- Has this company performed an analysis of its clay to identify the percentages of various minerals present?
- Has this clay undergone any tests to ensure purity? Does this clay meet the stringent USP/NF standards? (This may not be so important for some persons, as there are a few companies who sell good-quality clay, though unpurified.)

By now, you should be very familiar with the name *montmorillonite*. This is your clay of choice. But, if you see the name bentonite on a bottle, do not be so quick to set it down. Some companies use this name interchangably with *montmorillonite*. Read their literature to find out.

This leads us to the next step in choosing the right clay:

trial and errror. Just as with any other supplement in the health food store, some work for some people, and others don't. You may have to try a particular bottle of clay twice before you see any results. Or you may have to switch between different companies until you find a clay that you feel comfortable with. Be patient. This process of picking, choosing, and throwing away is entirely natural and is common in the natural health industry.

DIFFERENT SHAPES AND SIZES

Clay packaging comes in all different shapes and sizes. Some companies prefer to sell it as a powder, others in capsules, and still others in a liquid gel state. With so many forms to choose from, the following question naturally arises: Which clay is better to take internally?

The answer is that no method of packaging is superior to another. You will achieve the same results with any one you take. For instance, a liquid gel will act no differently than bulk powder. The entire matter is one of convenience and simply depends on your own preferences—that is, which is easier for you to take.

HOW AND WHEN TO TAKE IT

With capsules and pre-prepared liquid clay, the directions are already printed on the label. That will let you know how much to take and when to take it. When you purchase clay powder, on the other hand, it's a good idea to know what the average dose per person per day is.

Infants	1/4 to 1/2 teaspoon (in a bottle)
Small frame	one teaspoon

Medium frame	one heaping teaspoon
Large frame	one tablespoon
Extra large frame	one heaping tablespoon

Chapter 7 gave suggested dosages for each one of the listed ailments. Feel free to adjust the amount accordingly. If I suggested 3 teaspoons per day and you only need 2, then do whatever works for you. You can take as little as 1 teaspoon per day or as many as 20.

Independent experiments purposely designed to determine how much the clay's action would adversely affect the growth and health of experimental animals have indicated no ill effects when the intake did not exceed 25 percent of the total diet. If you have no special ailments and would like to take clay as a tonic and detoxifier, one to two doses per day is suggested.

Small Doses Are Better Than Big Doses

In a branch of natural medicine called homeopathy, ultra-small doses of certain medicines are given instead of mega-doses. That's because homeopathy is an energy medicine, and only a little bit of energy is needed to stimulate the energy of the immune system.

The same principle applies to clay. Generally speaking, the frequency of the dose is more important than the dose itself. Therefore, when you skip five days of clay and want to make up for it in one or two doses, remember that clay does not work that way. Its action is subtle in nature. It's better to take a little every day than a lot once in a while.

On an Empty Stomach

I find that clay works better when taken on an empty stomach so it can do its job freely and not be interfered with by digestion of food. It can be hard for clay to work while the intestinal tract is busy assimilating food.

Many people ask me what exactly an "empty stomach" means. I hope this helps:

- When you first wake up in the morning.
- At least one good hour before or after your meal. If you eat clay right before you eat food, the tendency is to get constipated.
- At night before you go to bed, providing you have not eaten for at least one hour.

Remember that clay can help with indigestion as well. Therefore, take it as needed—even if its right after a meal, or during a meal.

HOW TO STORE YOUR CLAY

You do not have to take any special precautions when storing clay. It is enough to keep it in dry, room-temperature conditions. If you would like to keep it on the kitchen counter or the pantry, this is okay. It need not be stored in the refrigerator.

Some people worry about leaving their clay in the sun, overnight in the car, or accidentally locked away in the dark. There is no problem with storing clay under any of these conditions. In fact, it is a good idea to keep your clay in contact with sunlight, perhaps letting it sit on the windowsill. Earlier when we talked about the cycle of the earth's growth, we referred to the clay receiving its energy from the sun and to its ability to potentially transfer that latent energy. Keeping the clay in contact with the sun is a good idea.

Clay can be stored for any length of time. Unlike vitamins and herbs, it does not lose potency, as minerals do not deteriorate with time.

WAYS TO PREPARE CLAY POWDER

Clay Water: This is the easiest drink to prepare. All you do is throw your clay in water (preferably distilled) and stir.

Muddy Mary: Put your clay in tomato juice. Serve at parties. The umbrella is optional.

Pile Driver: Clay in prune juice.

The Drainer: Clay with freshly squeezed lemon juice, barley greens, and psyllium seed powder.

Yodirt: For people who like to eat their clay as a sweet dessert. Add a teaspoon of clay and honey to yogurt and stir.

Mountain Meal: Clay with malto meal.

Clay Balls: Mix the clay with water and roll into tiny balls. Add a couple of drops of peppermint or tangerine essential oil for flavor, and set the balls out to dry. They make great candies to suck on.

Clay Chew: Add water to the clay to form a thick consistency. Then, as you wish, add a couple of drops of cinnamon or spearmint essential oil. Place a ball underneath your lip and allow it to dissolve. Don't worry about spitting it out; you can swallow it all.

Bibliography

Abehsera, Michael. *The Healing Clay*. Brooklyn, NY: Swan House Publishing, 1977, 1979.

Aninel, B., and S. Lagercrantz. *Geophagical Customs*. Uppsala: Almquist and Wiksells, Boktryckeri AB, 1958.

Anita, F. P. *Clinical Dietetics and Nutrition*. London: Oxford University Press, 1989.

Blatt, Harvey, Gerald Middleton, and Raymond Murray. *Origin of Sedimentary Rocks*. Englewood Cliffs, NJ: Prentice-Hall, 1972.

Clark, Linda. *Know Your Nutrition*. New Canaan, CT: Keats Publishing, 1973.

Damrau, Frederic. "The Value of Bentonite for Diarrhea." *Medical Annals of the District of Columbia* 30, No. 6 (June 1961): 326–328.

Degens, Egan T. *Geochemistry of Sediments: A Brief Survey*. Englewood Cliffs, NJ: Prentice-Hall, 1965.

Dextreit, Raymond. *Our Earth Our Cure*. New York: Carol Publishing Group, 1993.

Dunkel, Tom. "U.S. Unready for Viral Invasion." *Insight* (October 11, 1993).

Fairshter, Ronald D., and Archie F. Wilson. "Paraquat Poisoning: Manifestations and Therapy." *American Journal of Medicine* 59, No. 6 (December 1975): 751–753.

Gibson, Sheila, and Robin Gibson. *Homeopathy for Everyone*. Harmondsworth, England: Arkana, 1987.

Grim, Ralph E. *Applied Clay Mineralogy*. New York: McGraw-Hill, 1962.

———. "Clay Mineralogy." *Science* 135 (March 1962).

Heyman, Edward W., and Gerald Hartman. "Geophagy in Moustached Tamarins, Saguins Mystax (Platyrrhini: Callitrichidae), at the Rio Blanco, Peruvian Amazonia." *Primates* 32, No. 4 (October 1991): 533–537.

Homeopathy News & Views [Editorial] 94, No. 9 (September 1994).

Hunter, John M., and Oscar H. Horst. "Religious Geophagy As a Cottage Industry: The Holy Clay Tablets of Esquipulas, Guatemala." *National Geographic Research* 5, No. 3 (1989): 281–295.

Jensen, Neva. *The Healing Power of Living Clay*. Self-published, 1982.

Johns, Timothy, and Martin Duquette. "Detoxification and Mineral Supplementation As Functions of Geophagy." *American Journal of Clinical Nutrition* 53 No. 2 (February 1991): 448–456.

Jones, Robert L., and Harold C. Hanson. *Mineral Licks, Geophagy, and Biogeochemistry of North American Ungulates*. Ames, IA: State University Press, 1985.

Laufer, Berthold. *Geophagy*. Field Museum of Natural History, Publication 280, Anthropological Series Volume XVIII, No. 2. Chicago: 1980.

Lei, Lauana. "A Simple $10 Clay Bath Removes Toxic Metals and Chemicals from the Body." *The Awareness Journal* 3, No. 10 (July 1996): 7–16.

Lemonick, Michael D. "The Killers All Around." *Time* (September 12, 1994): 62–69.

Lipson, Steven M., and G. Stolzky. "Specificity of Virus Adsorption to Clay Minerals." *Canadian Journal of Microbiology* 31 (1985): 1–6.

Millot, Georges. "Clay." *Scientific American* 240 (April 1979): 109–118.

———. *Geology of Clays*. London: Chapman & Hall, 1970.

Mowrey, Daniel B. *The Scientific Validation of Herbal Medicine*. New Canaan, CT: Keats Publishing, 1990.

Powell, Eric F. W. *Health from the Earth, Air and Water*. N. Devon, UK: Health Science Press, 1970.

Robertson, Robert H. S. *Fuller's Earth: A History of Calcium Montmorillonite*. Hythe, UK: Volturna Press, 1986.

Sieskind, Odette. *Contribution to the Study of the Interactions of Clay and Organic Matter Adsorption of Amino Acids by Montmorillonite*. Strasbourg: Université de Strasbourg, 1962.

Tilden, John. *Toxemia: The Basic Cause of Disease*. Chicago: Natural Hygiene Press, 1974.

U.S. Office of Civil and Defense Mobilization. *Clay Masonry Family Fallout Shelters*. Washington, DC: Office of Civil and Defense Mobilization, 1960.

Walker, Norman. *Colon Health: The Key to a Vibrant Life*. Phoenix, AZ: O'Sullivan Woodside and Company, 1979.

Woods, Mike. "Infectious Ills Make Comeback." *The Arizona Republic* (August 15, 1993): A1–A2.

Resources

The following is a list of manufacturers who distribute clay products for internal use. Because so many companies produce clay for external use, their names are not included here. Products used externally include clay masks, ointments, soaps, and shampoos; they can be found in most health-food stores and some mass-market retail outlets. Products taken internally include pure clay supplements as well as those that contain a portion of clay in their supplement combination. If you plan to take therapeutic doses of clay, the pure clay supplements will be your best choice. The combination supplements that include clay typically contain very little—they are valuable insofar as the clay is synergistically combined with other ingredients. Read the label to get a pretty good idea of the amount of clay in the combination—and whether that amount will suit your needs.

Should you have diffficulty locating any of them, feel free to call or write to the company. Needless to say, the list does not contain every clay manufacturer because I am not familiar with all the smaller local companies. I encourage you to ask questions, be discriminating, and search for the product that best fits your needs. Good luck!

Arise N Shine
P.O. Box 1439
Mount Shasta, CA 96067
(800) 688-2444
Liquid Bentonite

Good N Natural
90 Orville Drive
Bohemia, NY 11716
(800) 544-0095

Natureade
7110 Jackson Street
Paramount, CA 90723
(562) 531-8120
(800) 367-2880
Colon Condition, available
   in tablets and powder

Nutraceutical Corporation
P.O. Box 681869
Park City, UT 84068
(800) 669-8877
Clay & Herbs Blend

Perfect 7
P.O. Box 2277
Seal Beach, CA 90740
(714) 229-8866
Psyllium-Herbal Combination

ProNatural
6211-A West Howard Street
Niles, IL 60714
(847) 588-0900
(800) 555-7580
Luvos Healing Earth,
   encapsulated

Rainbow Light Nutritional
   System
P.O. Box 600
Santa Cruz, CA 95061
(408) 429-9089
(800) 635-1233

Sonne's Organic Foods, Inc.
P.O. Box 2205
Kansas City, MO 64162
(800) 544-8147
Sonne's #7 Detoxificant
   (liquid montmorillonite)

Spectrum Essentials
Petaluma, CA 94954
(800) 995-2705
Daily Essential Fiber

Weider Nutrition
1960 S. 4250 West
Salt Lake City, UT 84204
(801) 975-5000
(800) 453-9542

Schiff product line, Dolomite
    powder, Tru-Dent
    toothpaste

White Rock Mineral
    Corporation
1130 South 350 East
Provo, UT 84606
(888) 328-2529

Yerba Prima, Inc.
740 Jefferson Avenue
Ashland, OR 97520
(541) 488-2228
(800) 488-4339
Great Plains Bentonite,
    Woman's Renew

Zand Herbal Formulas
P.O. Box 2039
Boulder, CO 80306
(800) 371-8420
Cleansing Fiber, Cleansing
    Laxative, Calcium &
    Magnesium Formula,
    Quick Cleanse Program